THE MYTH OF THE PERFECT MOM

THE MYTH OF THE PERFECT MOM

From Postpartum Perfection to Everyday Joy

ERIN SCHLOZMAN

alcove press

Books should be disposed of and recycled according to local requirements.
All paper materials used are FSC compliant.

Published in the United States by Alcove Press, an imprint of
The Quick Brown Fox & Company LLC.

Alcove Press and its logo are trademarks of
The Quick Brown Fox & Company LLC.

Library of Congress Catalog-in-Publication data available upon request.

ISBN (hardcover): 979-8-89242-423-3
ISBN (paperback): 979-8-89242-424-0
ISBN (ebook): 979-8-89242-425-7

Cover design by Hayley Warnham

Printed in the United States.

www.alcovepress.com

Alcove Press
34 West 27th St., 10th Floor
New York, NY 10001

First Edition: April 2026

The authorized representative in the EU for product safety and compliance
is eucomply OÜPärnu mnt 139b-14, 11317 Tallinn, Estonia,
hello@eucompliancepartner.com, +33757690241

10 9 8 7 6 5 4 3 2 1

To my mom, who has taught me
to be a mom.

To my Jack and Ruby, who made
me a mom.

To my husband, Richie, who continues to tell
me that the world deserves my work
and insists that I create.

And to my sister, Sarah, who has walked
beside me as we raise our babies together.

I can only take partial credit for this work,
and the rest belongs to you.

CONTENTS

INTRODUCTION

Stepping Into Motherhood

I became a mom to a little boy, Jack, in 2017 and a little lady, Ruby, born in the spring of 2020. After Jack was born, I was confident that I had postpartum figured out. I knew I could meet my baby's needs, and when I saw his beautiful little face for the first time, I was ready to pour all my energy into this new chapter of life. And if you had asked me in those early weeks of parenthood how I felt as a new mom, I would have told you that I loved it, it was easy, that I had finally found my life's one purpose and that becoming a mom was all I'd ever dreamed of. I would have told you that, and it would have been the biggest, boldest, and most beautiful lie.

The truth was, when I became a mom, everything changed: my priorities, my ambition, my sense of self. And as I tried to navigate all the life changes, it became painfully clear to me that society expected me to scale an absolutely impossible mountain. Not just to care for and love my baby but to do it flawlessly, perfectly, and with a smile. I had to be the best mom, the happiest mom, the perfect mom. But instead of feeling that bliss, I cried a lot, didn't think I was doing well enough, and wondered how anyone in the history of forever had been perfect at postpartum.

In all areas of my life, I had been high achieving: I had finished graduate school with a 4.0 GPA, passed board exams, obtained my clinical license, gotten a great job, married a wonderful man, and by all standards I was in the perfect place in life to have a baby. But when Jack was born, all I did was worry, panic, and then start Zoloft for the first time in my life, at thirty-three years old. I thought this meant I had already failed. And at two weeks postpartum, I found myself sitting cross-legged in the shower crying.

Are you nodding your head in agreement? Then you're in the right place.

Let me take a moment to introduce myself. I'm Erin, the mom and licensed therapist behind Erin Levin Counseling and the Instagram account 4th Trimester Wellness. My house is never as clean as I'd like it to be. Every week I pretend that this is going to be the week I start going back to Pilates. I wrote the majority of this book during nap time, middle-of-the-night quiet time, and early, early mornings watching the seasons come and go. I love being a mom, and the learning curve into motherhood was *nothing* I could have anticipated.

I have been working with new moms in a variety of settings, as a therapist, for the last ten-plus years. I started my career in community mental health, mainly driving people to and from a methadone clinic. I then worked at a psychiatric hospital as the primary therapist on the dual diagnosis and substance use disorder units. After the hospital, I became the lead clinician in a community crisis center, then the behavioral health provider on an addiction medicine team, then a corporate management consultant. I've worked with low-income moms, high-income moms, and everything in between.

While I was a corporate management consultant, I started 4th Trimester Wellness on Instagram, and a little further down the road the podcast *I Love My Baby, And . . .* We were in the middle of COVID, I had a new baby and understood the realities of how isolated new moms were feeling, and I wanted to be able to offer even the tiniest bit of comfort and support.

When I opened my private therapy practice in 2018, my focus was singular: Support pregnant and postpartum moms. That was it. Support the transition into motherhood, support the growing pains of new motherhood, be a safe space for postpartum moms.

Postpartum is a medical term to describe the period of time after the birth of a baby. I titled my business 4th Trimester Wellness because the "fourth trimester," a term coined by Dr. Harvey Karp in his book *Happiest Baby on the Block*, describes the postpartum period as spanning from baby's birth until they turn three months old. In my private practice and in my work, I follow this rule about the definition of postpartum: If you've had a baby, you are postpartum. You may be in your immediate postpartum, or you may be the parent of a toddler, but you'll always be in the period of time after birth and therefore postpartum.

There are three medical stages to the postpartum period: the *initial or acute postpartum* stage, the period six to eighteen hours after birth, where the birthing person can experience the most medical crises; the *subacute postpartum* stage, or up to two to six weeks after birth, when the birthing person is in recovery and still closely monitored; and the *delayed postpartum* stage, up to six months after birth.

If you're reading this and wondering if any of this information will apply to you—*Am I still considered postpartum? How long is the postpartum period?*—let me ease your mind first by telling you one of my favorite little tidbits: Postpartum is forever. Once you're a mom, you're a mom, and that can't be taken away from you. And the information in this book will help you with that transition into motherhood and beyond.

As my practice grew, I started to identify who was landing in my office and why. And behind closed doors, in the privacy of the therapy space, I heard, over and over, the trials of new moms who were used to being perfect and were struggling in their transition into motherhood. I have witnessed the profound impact that becoming a mother has on a woman's identity and have also witnessed how intense and painful postpartum can be when a new mom is expecting perfection.

Since that first day that I cried in the shower, I have sat with countless postpartum moms who are crying the same tears I cried. The moms who expect perfection from themselves. The moms who are shell-shocked by how much life changes when you step into motherhood. Touched-out moms, overstimulated moms, sad moms, angry moms. Moms who are starting to realize there is too much expected of them, recognizing either the unrealistic expectations they set for themselves or that the systems we live in aren't set up to support new moms.

Postpartum moms do a lot of caretaking. We clean up messy diapers, feed the baby constantly, keep the mood calm, and keep the house clean-ish. And if we complain about our role or new baby, it's only behind closed doors with our closest peers; otherwise, we keep our discomforts about the role to ourselves. We talk a lot about the baby. Everyone talks about the baby. Are they good sleepers? What color are their eyes? Are they good eaters? We talk about the baby, but we don't talk about whether the mom is okay—because keeping the secrets of postpartum is the unspoken arrangement women throughout history have upheld.

We are great at telling moms, especially new moms, *You have a new job now, and it's simple. Your new title is* Mom. *Maybe* Mama, *maybe* Mommy. *This new job title shall rule your whole life. You must gush about how amazing your two-month-old boss is, you can never complain about long hours or middle-of-the-night meetings, and you must continue to pursue one goal: be the mommiest of moms with no other goals, aspirations, or distractions.*

One of the most misunderstood aspects of motherhood is the idea that once a baby is born, we're supposed to know exactly what we're doing—and we need to do it with a smile. Or at least that's what the myth of perfection tells us. And this is where we do new moms a disservice.

When you're feeling lost in the newness of life with a baby, let this book be your guide. We'll work together to move your goalpost from striving for postpartum perfection to knowing you're accomplishing something great because you continue to show up each day with love in your heart. Your ability to dive into and live in the murkiness of postpartum life while caring for yourself, your baby, your body, your authenticity—this is where great moms are made. I know this because I've lived it. I learned the hard way that my love and my effort are my gifts to give. The rest didn't matter.

Many of us have been taught, however subtly, that our greatest accomplishments and proudest moments will be in finding a worthy partner and then having a baby. Educational degrees, moves, and career growth along the way are mere pit stops to the goals set by society: love, marriage, and baby.

And then, when the baby is born, we aren't often encouraged to create meaning in our lives outside of motherhood. Somewhere along the way, we have lost sight of the fact that motherhood is as much about the birth of a mom as it is about the baby. Becoming a mom isn't defined solely by big, celebratory, milestone moments: first steps, first words, first days of school. It's the early-morning snuggles when you're too tired to function. It's the quiet, chaotic routine of changing diapers, wiping noses, and folding endless loads of laundry. It's the quick, stolen moments of peace when your child finally falls asleep, and it's realizing at the end of the day that you're proud of yourself and that maybe, just maybe, you're doing a good job.

These small, often unnoticed moments are what make up the bulk, and the magic, of motherhood. The beauty and challenge of motherhood lives in the day-to-day, in the mundane, in the moments that don't make it into social feeds or shared family photo albums. Motherhood is full of contradictions. It's a love that feels infinite and overwhelming accompanied by a longing for space and time to yourself. It's pride in watching your child grow mixed with the bittersweet realization that they need you a little less each day. It's feeling powerful and capable while simultaneously questioning if you're doing anything right.

And when we focus on milestones rather than the postpartum moments we love, we fall into a trap of assuming that moms must be, and want to be, perfect.

But I'm happy to share that the perfect mom doesn't exist, and we can dismantle the myths we are taught about being the perfect mom.

You don't have to aim for perfection, you don't have to admire perfection, and you don't have to chase an unattainable goal of doing everything right. Life is far more complicated than giving birth to a baby and then everything after is a fairy tale. We are dynamic, and motherhood, especially postpartum, is also dynamic.

The Myth of the Perfect Mom is a book that calls for authenticity. It's about recognizing that the most fulfilling path in motherhood is one paved with self-acceptance, compassion, and the courage to redefine what it means to be a "good" mom.

Changing the Postpartum Narrative

"Isn't motherhood the best journey?" a stranger once asked me, her smile wide with curiosity. I was standing in the middle of a Denver sidewalk, holding a screaming newborn who hated his car seat while trying to put away a stroller I couldn't remember how to fold down. I was in my husband's sweats, hair in the highest bun I could muster, and all I wanted was to go home. Instead, a bright-eyed stranger was insisting on a philosophical conversation about the majesty of motherhood.

"Isn't motherhood the best journey?" she repeated, as if willing me to agree.

"Motherhood isn't a journey," I snarled back at her.

At the time, I didn't have the words to explain why her question got under my skin. Now, years later, I do.

When I think of a journey, I think of a beginning, middle, and end. A neat, clear progression from point A to point B. Maybe the path gets rocky, but it's still a path—something well worn, predictable, and navigable. Motherhood, though, is not any of those things. It's not a tidy sequence of milestones or a trail you can follow by reading someone else's map. Motherhood feels more like a labyrinth, or a Halloween corn maze that's grown too tall to see over. It's an explosion of love and exhaustion, joy and heartbreak. It's a renegotiation of everything you thought you knew about yourself and your life. It's constantly changing, it's unpredictable, and it's magic.

Motherhood isn't linear, like a walk in the woods. Nothing in life is linear. A journey suggests a starting point, specific milestones, and an eventual destination. Calling motherhood a journey implies that, along the way, a mother will progress, learn, grow, and ultimately arrive at some imagined end where she has everything perfectly figured out, where she has become the best, most perfect mother. And while there's beauty in this sentiment, it's not the reality of parenthood. Motherhood is something far more intricate, evolving, and personal.

Rather than seeing motherhood as a journey with the set destination of being a "good" or "perfect" mom, I think of it as a constant state of *becoming.* Every day, we are becoming something new. Some days we become more patient, more compassionate. Other days we become more tired, more lost, or more confused. We become excellent at shape-shifting in response to the needs of our children, our family, our circumstances, and ourselves. When we frame motherhood as an experience of becoming instead of a journey with a destination, we allow ourselves to see motherhood more as an ongoing process of self-discovery than it is reaching a specific and vague endpoint. It's messy, it's fluid, and it's ever-changing. And that's okay.

Telling a new mom "You wanted this, so you should be able to figure it out" isn't a great mantra for the new mom grasping for support. The myth that we were born to mother, so we should be great at it, reduces our experience in motherhood to a set of responsibilities or expectations, and it overlooks something much deeper: Motherhood, at its core, is about becoming; it's about being in relation.

Motherhood is not about how well you perform your duties or check tasks off your to-do list. It's about the unique, ever-changing relationship you share with yourself, with your child, and with the world around you. Sometimes this becomes close and connected; other times it's distant and strained. And that's normal. Like any relationship, our relationship with the role of motherhood requires attention, flexibility, and care. When we frame motherhood as a process of becoming rather than a journey, we let go of the pressure to "do" motherhood a certain way. Instead, we focus on building and nurturing a bond that is imperfect but real. Relationships don't have clear guidelines, and neither does motherhood. It's a dynamic, living connection that grows and shifts as you and your child grow.

Motherhood will never be a singular experience. It doesn't look or feel the same for everyone. It's deeply individual, shaped by personal circumstances, cultural backgrounds, and a lifetime of moments already lived. For some, motherhood might feel natural and fulfilling from day one. For others, it's an uphill battle of exhaustion, guilt, and self-doubt. Motherhood is joy and frustration, love and exhaustion, pride and uncertainty—all at once. And what would happen if we allowed ourselves to find ourselves in the good moments and the bad moments?

You don't have to fit into one narrative or follow a specific path to be a good mom. You just have to be you, as imperfectly authentic as you can be. That is the greatest gift you can give to both yourself and your baby.

How This Book Will Bust the Myth of a Perfect Postpartum

I know that the ingrained messages and standards that I've held myself to have at times held me back from being my most authentic self. I've been the perfectionist mom wanting to do everything right, driven by an unwavering desire for excellence. I've been the mom striving for impeccable outcomes in all aspects of my life, including motherhood. And I've learned that the relentless pursuit of perfection can lead to burnout, dissatisfaction, and disappointment. I've been the mom rocking her new baby in their gorgeous nursery while scrolling social media looking for solutions to the very natural challenges of early motherhood. I've had unrealistically high standards, periods littered with self-criticism, and, as hard as this is to admit, a deep desire to control every outcome.

I've also been an ambitious mom wanting validation. I've been fueled by an unstoppable drive and passion for both personal and professional success. I've embraced times where I thrive on the challenge of balancing motherhood with my own personal aspirations. I've juggled conference calls with nap time schedules and have prided myself on being a masterful multitasker, appearing totally competent to everyone around me. I've also been an ambitious mom who struggles with her work-life balance and the stigma that surrounds being a mom with career goals.

Maybe you're an ambitious first-time mom who wants to do everything right—but you're struggling with the burnout and exhaustion of the high standards society holds for what it means to be a mother. This book is for you.

Maybe you're a people-pleasing mom who spends each day trying to make sure everyone around you is well kept while also completely neglecting your own needs. Perhaps you've even gone so deep into pleasing your people that you've lost sight of who you are and what you need. This book is for you.

Maybe you're postpartum with your second, third, or fourth child and you feel your fire is completely gone. You don't recognize who you've become or what motivates you. You're chronically tired, chronically online, and chronically feeling like your attention is so split that nobody gets the best version of you, just the fractured version. This book is also for you.

Maybe you're a postpartum mom who's feeling like something isn't right. You love your baby and are longing for more. You're staying home and finding it less fulfilling than you expected. You've returned to work and are finding it less fulfilling than you expected. You're feeling lonely but don't want or know how to find your village. If you're a postpartum mom and want reassurance, validation, and for someone to remind you how well you're *already* doing, this book is for you.

In each chapter of *The Myth of a Perfect Mom*, I take aim at the biggest culprits: the myths that I see showing up for new moms the most often, myths that we can free ourselves from. At the end of each chapter, you will find a set of activities—in a section I call the Road Map to Change—that will allow you to take a closer look at how the myth we've just discussed is showing up in your life. I give you a variety of tools you can easily implement to change your mindset. I recommend getting a new note started in your notes app, or pull out your favorite journal—these are perfect places to track your own growth by jotting down ideas you love and starring parts you want to return to. You will find each road map attainable, actionable, and easy to follow, and you can return to it anytime you need.

In each chapter I will share pieces of my own story, but you will also get to read the stories of other postpartum moms who came to see me for therapy, each bringing their own struggles, successes, and postpartum experiences. Throughout this book, postpartum will be the thread that connects all of us. I bet, in each of these personal stories, you will find a bit of yourself. We'll look at a little history, a little cultural background that explains how we've gotten to this place of thinking that perfection and postpartum are besties, and we'll tackle one myth at a time so that you can have the best introduction into motherhood possible. It won't be easy, but I promise it will be worth it.

Here's your road map to each chapter. In **Chapter 1: The Myth of the Perfect Mom**, we explore where striving for postpartum perfection comes from and how it has become so incredibly engrained in the ethos of motherhood. Then, in **Chapter 2: The Myth of the Perfect Birth**, we look at our own biases around birthing, birth trauma, and how to work through our own feelings about our birth stories. A lot of birthing experiences exist outside of intervention-free births, and we deserve to feel empowered by our births regardless of how the baby came out.

In **Chapter 3: The Myth of the Perfect Way to Feed Your Baby**, we dive into how moms can't win with feeding expectations. We explore the stigmas surrounding how a mom chooses to feed her baby and uncover tools that will help you love your feeding experience—no matter what it looks like.

In **Chapter 4: The Myth of the Perfectly Innate Mother**, we learn the differences between natural instincts and the learned art of mothering. Becoming a mom is more than just knowing what to do; it's also about learning what to do. And in **Chapter 5: The Myth of the Perfect Mom-Baby Attachment**, I'll clear up the question of attachment, which can be *so* confusing. How do we form it, when do we know we have it, and why is it important? We are going to dive deep into attachment theory in ways that are accessible—you deserve to understand how and why we attach the way we do.

In **Chapter 6: The Myth of "Mom" Being Your Only Identity**, I remind you that having a baby doesn't mean you're a completely different person than you were nine months ago, but it does mean you have a newly added identity. We'll look at identity formation during the postpartum period.

Chapter 7: The Myth That Self-Sufficiency = Success in Postpartum attacks the commonly held idea that if you can't manage all of postpartum life alone, then you are unfit (in some made-up and pretend way, we've come to believe this). You're allowed to need help; it isn't natural to mother alone. Self-sufficiency is great, but it's also overrated.

Chapter 8: The Myth of the Perfect Postpartum Body addresses the myth that you must look, work, and live like you've never had a baby while simultaneously loving every moment of motherhood.

If you have any questions about postpartum mood disorders, **Chapter 9: The Myth of the Perfect Postpartum Mood** is where you'll find your answers. We'll look at common mood changes that happen with having a baby, and we'll look at perinatal mood disorders so you can feel empowered and on top of your mental health during such a crucial time.

Finally, in **Chapter 10: The Myth That Motherhood isn't Ambitious**, we scrutinize how ambition and motherhood are perceived. I personally feel that motherhood is the most ambitious thing any woman can do. Taking on the task of raising our next generation is no small feat, and tackling this role is far more ambitious than many of the career ladders we choose to climb.

As we dismantle the ten different myths of the perfect mom, I give you permission to say, "Screw it, I'm going to do this my way." These are the benefits you will see by dismantling these myths:

- **Increased self-acceptance and self-esteem**: When women feel comfortable being their true selves, they are more likely to accept and appreciate their unique qualities. This can lead to a boost in self-esteem and confidence.
- **Improved mental and emotional well-being**: Authentic expression can reduce stress, anxiety, and depression. It can also promote feelings of happiness, ease, and fulfillment.

- **Enhanced creativity and problem-solving:** When moms aren't bound by the expectations of others, they are free to explore their own ideas and perspectives. This can lead to increased creativity, innovation, and *fun* in parenthood.
- **Stronger relationships**: Authenticity fosters genuine connections with others, as it allows people to build relationships based on mutual respect and understanding. This is the first step to building a lifelong postpartum village.
- **A greater sense of purpose and meaning**: Living authentically can help people identify their true passions and values. This can lead to a greater sense of purpose and direction in their parenting experience.
- **Reduced fear of judgment**: When moms are authentic, they are less likely to be afraid of what others think of them. This can lead to a greater sense of freedom and liberation.

It's time we rewrite the script on perfectionism and postpartum. It's time we set ourselves free of the pressure to live up to impossible standards. It's time to allow postpartum moms to celebrate the learned art of nurturing and to embrace the ebbs and flows of growth and identity formation. We are allowed to claim a sense of pride in our bodies as being strong instead of broken. I want to celebrate the diversity of our motherhood experiences and honor the evolution of self. Your needs matter, your ambition matters, and the world deserves your most authentic self. This is your permission to radically embrace your own definitions of success in parenthood and to celebrate it.

And . . . the irony isn't lost on me that I'm writing a book about ditching perfection in motherhood, yet here I am, striving to write the perfect book. And that's the whole point. We win some, we lose some, but most importantly, we learn and share our experiences. That's the heart and soul of this book: to empower you to mother authentically, make your transition into parenthood meaningful, and finally, update the outdated language around the postpartum experience.

So, if you're tired of chasing perfection, if you're ready to embrace the beautiful messiness of motherhood, if you're yearning for a community that understands the roller coaster of emotions, the doubts, the triumphs, and everything in between—welcome. This book is for you. Let's journey together, imperfectly perfect, toward a postpartum experience that's filled with authenticity, joy, and the freedom to simply be ourselves.

1

The Myth of the Perfect Mom

A myth is a story or belief that history tells itself so often that it starts to feel like it's true. Myths become the framework that influences how we see ourselves and others, especially in the role of motherhood.

One example of a myth is *Babies are supposed to sleep through the night*. While this ideal is lovely, it is also completely untrue. Babies are supposed to wake at night: They get hungry, they need comfort, and they often need a two AM diaper change. That's the reality. So when someone tells me that their baby is sleeping through the night beautifully at three weeks old, I'm never surprised when the first sleep regression hits and that lovely pattern abruptly halts.

Another myth that I love: *Successful people are the ones who work the hardest and deserve their success*. This is also a beautiful ideal that is completely BS. First, everyone's measure of success is different, because we all want different things, especially postpartum, when we are figuring out what success even means. Also, success isn't just about hard work. It is influenced by luck, privilege, timing, and opportunity. A mom who has committed to being a stay-at-home mom is going to have a different idea of daily success than a mom who is running a board meeting after day care drop-off.

Culturally, we have widely accepted the myth of the perfect mom that tells us we should be endlessly patient, ever loving, always confident, and never wavering in our obsession for our new role as moms. This myth about motherhood shapes our expectations, sets invisible standards, and usually makes new moms feel like they aren't doing a good-enough job.

In the privacy of my therapy office, in the DMs of social media, and in texts between friends, I have had the privilege of hearing all about the lives of new parents: the high highs and the low lows. I've been privy to the struggles of contemporary mothers, often concealed behind the myth of perfection, which is the voice that makes moms second-guess their ability to parent. It's the urge to apologize when we don't know what we're apologizing for. The perfect-mom myth is a set of expectations of modern mothers that we've put on ourselves, and it tells us:

1. We must want to be a parent;
2. We must be the best parents;
3. We must love and uphold our new role as moms as our first and most important priority; and
4. We can't take up space, shine too bright, or rock the boat.

Yet, in those solitary moments, shielded from judgment, the fear of failing at motherhood occupies many moms' thoughts, feelings, and ability to explore what motherhood *could* be if they stopped focusing on what it *should* be.

Noticing that societal expectations about what postpartum should look like didn't match up with what I wanted it to be was my first step in breaking free of the myth of perfection. It allowed me to begin to reject these expectations and live more authentically.

One moment that stands out to me in my adjustment to authenticity was when I was four weeks postpartum with my first baby and I accepted an invitation to be the new-mom guest speaker for a group of expectant first-time moms. I was asked to share the "easy to digest" parts of my labor and delivery. As a therapist and new mom, I was familiar with this group and the therapist colleague who would be running the session. I said yes to being a guest for this group session despite oversupply that was leaking everywhere, ongoing C-section recovery, crippling anxiety, and not feeling like I was the "expert" new mom the group was promised. I was feeling more along the lines of a mom who had labored for thirty-six hours, pushed for four, then ended up with a C-section and was feeding using nipple shields. And still, because the "perfect mom" says yes, I, too, said yes. I had already begun navigating the pressure to perform and the pressure surrounding my own perfect-mom myth.

The therapist leading the session had older kids; she had moved through her early family-planning stage and her infant and toddler stages. She asked me, "Do you like being a mom?"

Me and my perfect-mom aspirations said, "Yes! It's the best." I had subconsciously decided that I needed to present myself as capable, rested, fully transitioned, and incredibly grateful for my new role as a mom. But what I really wanted to say was *Um, I think my baby's really cute, I think the hours are grueling, I don't know if I consider myself a mom yet, and my nipples feel like they're going to fall off. Also, my mom hasn't left yet because suddenly—after years of ultra independence—I don't like being alone*. For me, the reality was that caretaking and loving my baby had come quickly. But finding my identity and sense of self in this new role hadn't.

But I didn't say that. Instead, I gave the answer that I thought she wanted to hear, because I assumed everyone else would have gasped if I had been honest about my parenting experience.

I have met countless moms who love their babies and struggle with the weight of the "perfect mom" expectation. Expectations like *Don't work, but be ambitious*, *Don't get angry, Don't ask for or need help, Don't leave your partner sexually unsatisfied, Don't have opinions,* and *Never talk about being tired.*

Every mom has their own ingrained perfect-mom myth: Moms who are suffocating in the newborn stage and regretting their decision to have a baby but wait until they're in the privacy of the therapy office to talk about it. Moms who are experiencing unwanted intrusive thoughts and are too scared to talk about them for fear of what others may think. Any mom desperately looking for solutions to make early motherhood easier but not talking about it. That is the perfect-mom myth: the voice that tells us we can't be honest about our experiences because then we won't be "good."

Many new moms get stuck in loops of fear, and often what they had imagined early motherhood would be is far from the reality of day-to-day life with a baby, and they end up feeling lied to. As little girls, we are taught that if we're lucky, we'll be someone's mom and wife. Our current generation of moms has been told our whole lives that we can have it all: We can have a career, a family, and a house as well as travel. But we aren't told at what cost, and we aren't told that while we pile on the "having it all," there isn't going to be anyone taking anything off our already-crowded plates. We're free to have unlimited baggage, but nobody is going to help us carry it. So we either buck-up-buttercup or find a new way that works.

My client Sam was one of those mothers who felt the pressure to do it all.

Sam's Story

Sam came to meet me when she was four months postpartum with her third child. She was struggling in the most personal areas of her life: being a stay-at-home mom to three young kids, a partner with a demanding job limiting the amount of support she had at home, and the social pressures of feeling like she had to play an engaged role as a connector in her community. She was avoidant in her approach to therapy and seemed to have separated her sense of self from her new role as a mom to three. It took many sessions for her to find the words that connected her feelings to her experience.

"I should have this down by now; it's my third baby. I'm supposed to be good at this. I'm supposed to have it all handled, and I'm supposed to be enjoying it."

She described her days as a relentless attempt to check every box: engaging her kids educationally, nutritionally, and spiritually; keeping her house in perfect order; bonding with her baby while staying connected to her two older kids. Every night she went to sleep feeling like a failure. She woke up each morning dreading that she would fail again on the new day.

"I just can't keep up," she would tell me for many weeks, then many months. "If I can't do this right, what does this say about me as a mother?"

I asked Sam about how she was mothered as a young girl and about patterns of people-pleasing and perfection that I saw as a thread woven through each area of her story we explored. She had a profound and fundamental belief that if she only tried a little harder, she'd be able to do better.

I could see the cracks in her confidence. And from where I sat, she was doing a phenomenal job. I observed that her perfectionism had been driving her to parent from a place of constant tension and self-criticism, which, of course, left little room for joy or connection. Instead of allowing herself to be imperfect, she focused on controlling every detail around her, making her feel stuck in a maze.

One of my offerings in private practice is called walk-and-talk sessions. I meet a new mom at her house or a park near her house, and we go for a stroll. It can be easier to allow feelings out of a cage in the open air, and for some clients, getting out of the house with a newborn is the one barrier to therapy. Providing accessibility to therapy is important to me.

A few months into working with Sam, she scheduled a walk-and-talk session. Sam told me that she had lost all of her cool earlier that morning, screamed at her kids, and stormed out. She told me she felt mortified. This was the first time Sam didn't say she needed to *do better* but instead said, "Something has to change." I witnessed her address her myth of the perfect mom in real time. She was acknowledging that her pursuit of perfection was moving her further away from being the mom she wanted to be, and it was time for things to shift.

After this session, there was no single solution, easy strategy, or new, fresh approach for her to take to tackle her years of perfectionism. But she did leave the session with something else—a growing awareness that maybe her hard moments weren't failures and weren't even really problematic. She walked away with a slight understanding that she wasn't allowing herself to falter or be anything other than perfect and that this was the real culprit in her distress.

For every parent, the Perfect Mom Myth is its own unique cocktail (well, mocktail, unless you plan to pump and dump), with ingredients sourced from childhood experiences, friendships, and the combination of societal, religious, and historical factors that create a unique but somehow pervasive set of expectations about the standard of womanhood. And it impacts all of us. For Sam, it took her hitting a breaking point to realize that maybe she wasn't the problem but that societal expectations placed on modern mothers were the problem.

The perfect-mom myth creates a space that doesn't allow parents to explore the everyday reality that the complex parts of motherhood and the wonderful parts can exist together and that moms can speak on both without feeling ungrateful. I've heard, "I wanted this, so it's my responsibility to take on motherhood alone," too often. Aren't we allowed to want something and still be challenged by the experience?

Culturally, we've grown accustomed to viewing motherhood as an idealized image or aesthetic rather than recognizing it as the complex, emotional, and multifaceted milestone it is. Over the last hundred years, we have romanticized the role of motherhood as one that demands constant perfection, availability, and selflessness while also shouldering the lion's share of the emotional and domestic duties at home. We give no thought to recognizing motherhood as a profound shift in our mental, physical, and spiritual transformation from nonparent to parent.

The image of the "perfect mother" didn't appear overnight. Its roots come from a complex tapestry woven from historical, cultural, and religious threads, including evolving parenting ideals, shifting gender roles, media portrayals, and social movements. Watching other moms perform motherhood for the camera has perpetuated the idea that a "perfect mother" bounces back quickly, has time to exercise, and never has a messy car. Let's take a closer look at this complex tapestry and the history that got us to the perfect-mom myth.

Understanding the Stories We've Absorbed: The History of the Perfect-Mom Myth

We may not be able to pinpoint one exact moment in history when the myth of the perfect mom was born, but many historical and cultural contexts have contributed to its formation—and perpetuation. Over time, there has been an evolution of parenting ideals and different ways that history has shaped the role of "mom" in a complex intersection of religion, gender roles, media and literature influence, social movements, gender-based consumerism, and social expectation.

To understand how the myth of the perfect mom persists, we can look back to the nineteenth and twentieth centuries for trends and shifts in the way motherhood has been experienced and perceived. One of the most influential ideologies shaping expectations of mothers was the *cult of domesticity*, which emerged in the early nineteenth century. This belief system positioned women as the moral guardians of the home, responsible for raising virtuous children, supporting their husbands, and maintaining a pure and nurturing domestic space.

The phrase *cult of domesticity* first appeared in scholarly discussions in the mid-twentieth century, though the ideology it describes dates back to the early nineteenth century. Historian Barbara Welter is often credited with popularizing the term in her 1966 article "The Cult of True Womanhood: 1820–1860." In this work, she examined how nineteenth-century literature, sermons, and advice manuals promoted four key virtues for women: piety, purity, submissiveness, and domesticity.

Earlier discussions of similar ideas can be found in feminist writings from the late nineteenth and early twentieth centuries, such as those by Charlotte Perkins Gilman and Elizabeth Cady Stanton, who critiqued the idealization of women's domestic roles. However, the specific term *cult of domesticity* as a historical framework became widely recognized after Welter's work and has since been expanded upon by historians analyzing gender roles and women's history.

Piety refers to religious devotion and moral virtue. Women were expected to be the spiritual leaders of the household, nurturing religious faith and maintaining a moral environment at home. Piety was seen as a way for a woman to exert influence in the home, specifically through religion.

Purity emphasizes the importance of sexual modesty. Women were expected to remain sexually pure before marriage and to uphold high moral standards. During certain times in history, a woman's sexual purity was tied to a woman's worth, and deviating from this purity could damage her reputation and the reputation of her family. Today we can see this come into play when we talk about birthing practices and rituals around menstruation.

Submissiveness is the idea that women are expected to be obedient, passive, and deferential. This virtue reinforced the belief that a woman's role was supporting and following men's leadership, staying within a submissive and quiet sphere, particularly in matters outside the home.

Domesticity refers to a woman's primary role within the home, taking care of household duties like cleaning, cooking, and raising children. Domesticity frames women as caretakers and nurturers responsible for maintaining the home as a moral sanctuary.

The *cult of domesticity* wasn't just about what women *did*—it was about who they were supposed to be. The ideal mother was selfless, endlessly patient, and naturally attuned to her children's needs. Her identity revolved entirely around caregiving, and any personal ambition or struggle was seen as secondary—or even as a failure. While this ideal primarily applied to white, middle-class women, it influenced broader cultural norms, reinforcing the idea that a "good mother" was one who sacrificed everything for her family.

These expectations didn't disappear with time; they evolved. By the mid-twentieth century, the rise of psychology, child development theories, and consumer culture layered new pressures onto the old ideal. Mothers were no longer just responsible for their children's survival and moral upbringing—they were now expected to ensure their emotional well-being, cognitive development, and future success. The perfect mother was no longer just a devoted homemaker; she was also an expert in every aspect of child rearing, held to impossible standards that still shape modern motherhood today.

This messaging has, in many ways, remained the same over the span of a hundred years. Leta Hollingworth's 1916 article "Social Devices for Impelling Women to Bear and Rear Children" argued that motherhood had long been used as a tool of social control—keeping women docile, tied to childbearing, and confined to the home. Nearly a century later, a 2005 *Newsweek* feature titled "The Myth of the Perfect Mother" explored how social expectations had turned motherhood into an impossible performance, driven by unattainable ideals and the relentless pursuit of perfection.

Most recently, in August 2024, US surgeon general Dr. Vivek Murthy issued an advisory highlighting the significant stress and mental health challenges faced by parents, labeling it an urgent public health issue. The advisory emphasized that parents consistently reported higher stress levels compared to nonparents, with 33 percent of parents having experiencing high stress in the past month versus 20 percent of other adults. Additionally, 48 percent of parents felt their stress was overwhelming most days, compared to 26 percent of nonparents.

Despite the decades between them, these works build upon one another, revealing a persistent message: Women who prioritize any role outside of motherhood are seen as failing their families, while those who fully devote themselves to motherhood are held to impossible standards. No matter how much progress is made, the structures in place keep reinforcing the idea that a woman's primary duty is motherhood—and that any deviation from this role must be corrected.

Hollingworth asserts that societal structures are designed to keep women out of the workforce. For those who manage to break through barriers, there are mechanisms in place to push them back before they can gain real momentum. Even today, when a woman achieves the same level of success as her male counterparts, her accomplishments are often framed as a failure to prioritize her family.

Historically, we can see a long pattern of motherhood being used as a tool to seclude women from men—not only in public spaces such as work but also with enforced laws—and these historical imprints of seclusion feed into the myth of maternal perfection, suggesting that a perfect mother must be out of the public eye for the comfort of those around her. Whether on a micro scale or in the context of more considerable societal expectations, gender-based separations have not only impacted women in their homes but have also had a lasting impact on women's opportunities in education and employment, which reinforces the notion that women should remain in limited roles in public spaces. For example, my mom, who graduated from high school in 1972, was advised against pursuing higher education, believing that her job was to find a husband, not to get an advanced degree. This stance reflected a broader societal expectation that women's primary role should be in motherhood rather than personal or professional aspirations.

Such gender stereotypes and societal expectations significantly impact a woman's self-confidence and willingness to take up space, specifically to be anything other than "the perfect mom." This struggle for balance and recognition has been further compounded by the portrayal of women in media, literature, and art. As a millennial, I grew up in the height of young female pop stars—many of whom fell out of the limelight after going through puberty or having their kids. This validated the idea that we can't be seen if we're old, tired, or have had kids on the hip.

Again and again, I return to this subtle messaging: Instead of teaching girls that they hold immense power in their ability to bring life into the world, society treats women as liabilities *because* we have that ability.

Today, as new mothers navigate expectations around nurturing, availability, and emotion regulation, there remains a subtle but enduring belief that things moms experience—like burnout, the drain of the mental load and carrying the emotional labor of the family—should not be discussed. *Frontiers in Psychology* published a study in 2018 titled "Feeling Pressure to Be a Perfect

Mother Relates to Parental Burnout and Career Ambitions." This article states that "intense mothering norms prescribe women to be perfect mothers," finding that when women feel pressure to be the perfect mother, they have higher levels of parental burnout and parental stress and lower work-family balance relating to lower career ambitions.

Present-Day Pressure to Be Perfect

In America today, the expectation of perfection is everywhere: Give birth a certain way, look a certain way, have your house look a certain way, want to have sex, and be sexually appealing to your partner. Postpartum-bounce-back culture is an excellent example of how we link mothers to perfection by focusing on their physical appearance in relation to their worthiness. We are expected to have a baby without looking like we had a baby within weeks of having an actual human baby.

My client Ellie experienced this exact pressure—to be perfect before and after birth. Ellie came to see me for the first time when she was six months pregnant. There was a widening emotional and physical gap between her and her husband. "He hates my pregnant body. He won't touch me. I'm so hurt," she said during one of our first sessions.

As she continued to grow during her pregnancy, her husband became less affectionate, more disinterested, and "repulsed" by just the suggestion of having sex with her. This weighed heavily on Ellie. She was hurt and confused, as they had both been excited to welcome a baby, and now she was being made to feel othered by her husband's distaste for a pregnant woman looking pregnant. The fact was that the changes Ellie and her body were going through were totally normal.

When Ellie's partner expressed disinterest in her pregnant body, it tapped into deeply rooted stereotypes around femininity, motherhood, and the cultural expectations placed on modern moms.

Modern moms are standing on years and years of generational conditioning in which, from a young age, we are taught to be polite, demure, and accommodating, reinforcing the idea that being a desired woman is among the most important virtues a woman can hold.

Even after their baby was born, Ellie struggled with the lingering effects of those months of rejection. The unspoken message—that her worth was tied to her desirability—didn't fade just because she was no longer pregnant. Instead, it morphed into a new set of impossible expectations: She was now supposed to "bounce back," to erase the visible evidence of childbirth as quickly as possible, all while being a devoted and selfless mother.

This is the trap of the perfect-mom myth. Women are told that motherhood should be all-consuming, yet they are also expected to maintain an effortless attractiveness. They must give everything to their child while somehow remaining unchanged—still sexy, still accommodating, still fitting within the narrow definitions of desirability that existed before they became mothers.

Ellie's experience is not uncommon. Many new moms find themselves caught between these conflicting demands, feeling as though they are failing no matter what they do. If they prioritize their baby, they risk losing their sense of self—or, as Ellie experienced, their partner's attraction. If they prioritize themselves, they risk being seen as selfish or not maternal enough.

The myth of the perfect mom thrives in these contradictions, setting women up to feel inadequate at every turn. But Ellie's story also reveals the power of awareness and conversation. By naming these impossible standards, we can begin to dismantle them—giving women permission to exist in their evolving bodies without shame, to embrace motherhood without erasure, and to be seen as whole people, not just as ideals to be maintained.

The rise of the modern momfluencer, and its constant stream of curated images and stories, has not helped mothers feel less inadequate. Such constant exposure to this idealized variety of motherhood exacerbates the pressure to be perfect. Although well meaning, the rise of the momfluencer has reinforced perpetuating gender stereotypes, demonstrated a lack of diversity and representation, and promoted consumption as a way to be the perfect mom.

Do I want to be able to have all the fun cleaning gadgets that momfluencers are sharing? Possibly, yes. Do I have the time to make a goo ball for cleaning out the nooks and crannies of my car? Absolutely not. A simple scroll through social media can demonstrate the popularization of two types of moms: the hot-mess mom and the picture-perfect mom. And, as to be expected, anything less than the perfect mom makes you the hot-mess mom: always running late, always missing a diaper, always unshowered with a messy bun. This binary division creates an environment of judgment and pressure for moms to fit into one of these categories. Still, the reality is that a lot exists between hot mess and the Pinterest-perfect mom. And this is the space that most modern moms live in.

As mothers, we often sacrifice our own desires and needs for the greater good of the people around us because we think we have to. Perfectionism stifles modern moms' rich, complex, and beautifully imperfect identity, denying them the space to be their authentic selves among the unrealistic ideals we've created. It's high time we tore down these myths, freeing moms to define motherhood on their terms and allowing them to feel their feelings.

Historical perspectives of the perfect mom have evolved with the development of attachment theories, parenting books, and the rise of the mommy influencer: a little more "you need to know" with a little less "you need to be physically attractive" with a lot of pressure to be perfect, even when perfection comes at a high cost.

Let's look a little closer at how the ideals of the perfect mom have changed and evolved.

The Evolution and Stagnation of the Myth of the Perfect Mom

The ideal of the "perfect mom" is both ever changing and stubbornly unshakable. On the surface, motherhood today looks vastly different from the way it did in past generations—women now have greater access to education, careers, and reproductive choices. Yet despite these shifts, the core expectations of motherhood remain strikingly similar. Mothers are still held to impossibly high standards, expected to be selfless, nurturing, and wholly dedicated to their children while balancing societal pressures to maintain an idealized version of womanhood.

How the Ideal of the Perfect Mom Hasn't Changed Over Time

1. **Self-sacrifice:** The idea that a mother should prioritize her children above all else has remained the same. Mothers are still expected to be selfless, placing their needs at the bottom of the priority list, secondary to their family's well-being.
2. **Emotional availability:** From historical expectations of gentle and nurturing mothers to the present-day ideal of emotionally attuned, empathic parenting, the demand for motherhood to provide emotional availability remains steady.

3. **The moral compass:** Historically, mothers have been viewed as moral role models for their children and responsible for instilling values, and today, mothers are still expected to make sure this happens.
4. **Home as the priority:** Regardless of additional responsibilities or personal aspirations, society still expects mothers to be the main organizers of the household. Whether hosting, cleaning, or creating and maintaining a welcoming environment, the connection between motherhood and homemaking remains strong.
5. **The emotionally regulated and the emotional regulator:** Patience has been a hallmark of the idealized mom forever. Historical and modern expectations demand that mothers keep their emotions in check, avoiding outward displays of frustration, anger, or stress. Mothers today are still judged by their ability to "stay calm" in challenging moments.

How Ideals of the Perfect Mother Have Changed Over Time

1. **Recognition of individual identity:** In the past, a woman's identity was often seen as her role in the family—a mother. Today there's a greater recognition that women are individuals with dynamic needs, goals, and aspirations outside of parenting. This shift acknowledges that motherhood is part of a woman's life rather than her entire identity, encouraging mothers to pursue personal ambitions alongside their family commitments.
2. **Mental health support:** Unlike previous generations of mothers, we have made great headway in understanding the mental health challenges of being a modern mother. Open conversations about maternal mental health are

being destigmatized, providing modern moms with better access to support, resources, and therapeutic validation.

3. **Emphasis on partnered parenting:** The modern ideal places less pressure on mothers to be the sole caretakers, and dads and partners are being praised for their involvement in domestic labor. This shift emphasizes coparenting as a new norm and encourages a more equitable distribution of tasks, emotional support, household management, and responsibilities.
4. **Conversations around self-care:** Today we are creating space for moms to prioritize self-care practices as well as hobbies and interests unrelated to their kids. This move is helping to shift the focus away from motherhood as a purely self-sacrificing endeavor and to normalize teaching new moms that self-care is not selfish but necessary for sustainable and healthy parenting.
5. **Flexible parenting styles:** Modern motherhood is more accepting of diverse parenting approaches, recognizing that every mother and every child is different, with a unique set of needs.

These positive changes have undoubtedly fostered a more inclusive and supportive environment for postpartum moms, and I appreciate that these changes demonstrate the many nuances of modern parenting. But modern moms are still climbing uphill to beat their perfectionism.

I'm so excited to present to you our first Road Map to Change: practicing imperfection, on purpose.

Road Map to Change: The Practice of Imperfection

Welcome to your first Road Map to Change. We first look a little more closely at how you can "practice" imperfection, and

I follow it up with some exercises that reinforce those learnings. With all these tools, take baby steps. Start with small, manageable bits. Keep a journal to clarify what you want to work on and how you will do it. It's easy as a mom to steamroll through the day; some days, that alone is a huge success. We're working toward flexibility, not perfection. And remember, we are working on taking baby steps to ease into our own breakup with perfectionism.

First and foremost, *you deserve the benefits of not being perfect.* It feels very counterintuitive to stop striving for perfection, but let's look at the benefits of practicing imperfection in motherhood, and you may change your mind. Also, with the moms I work with in my office, I like to replace the word *imperfect* with the word *flexibility.*

Focusing on flexibility allows us to shift our focus from unattainable and rigid standards to more realistic, adaptable expectations. Think about flying a kite. When we hold on tightly, we'll get flung around. But when we hold a kite with a loose grip, we allow the kite to do what it will do while also staying grounded. And remember, *you are flexible*; you're already practicing being flexible. That's what postpartum is, a big practice in flexibility. You can handle many roles and many responsibilities in different ways and still get what you need to get done accomplished.

The Power of Flexibility in Motherhood

Motherhood is often framed as a path with rigid rules and clear right and wrong choices. But the reality is far more complex—every child, every family, and every circumstance is different. Embracing flexibility isn't about lowering standards or "giving up"; it's about adapting, making room for nuance, and recognizing that there is no single right way to parent.

Practicing flexibility benefits not only individual mothers but also society as a whole. On a personal level, it allows moms to release the guilt and pressure of perfection, fostering resilience, confidence, and emotional well-being. On a broader scale, when flexibility is embraced collectively, it challenges outdated norms, supports more equitable parenting roles, and creates a culture that values diverse approaches to raising children.

Both the individual and societal benefits of practicing flexibility in motherhood can lead to healthier, happier moms and a more supportive world for families. Some of the individual benefits include:

1. **Reduced stress and anxiety:** When we accept that imperfection is inevitable and even normal, we can let go of some of that pressure and reduce stress and anxiety.
2. **Increased self-compassion:** It becomes easier to be compassionate toward ourselves when we learn to accept our flaws and mistakes. This can lead to a more positive self-image and increased self-esteem.
3. **Greater resilience:** When we face challenges and setbacks, we are more likely to bounce back if we believe that we are not failures just because we are not perfect.
4. **Enhanced creativity and innovation:** Perfectionism can stifle creativity and innovation because it discourages experimentation and risk-taking. When we embrace imperfection, we are more open to trying new things and exploring new possibilities and in turn having the parenting experience we want.
5. **More authentic relationships:** When we are true to ourselves and accept our imperfections, it allows us to build deeper and more authentic relationships with others. When "impressing" others isn't our top priority, we get to welcome increased authenticity in our relationships instead. I love that for all of us.

Some societal benefits of flexibility include:

1. **More realistic expectations:** Having realistic expectations in motherhood is crucial for our personal and professional wellness. For example, take the expectation that the house will be spotless all of the time after the baby arrives. Realistically, newborns require constant care and energy is limited. The idea that a new mom should maintain the same level of household productivity as before is unrealistic. These are instances when "good enough" is actually, truly, good enough.
2. **Increased diversity and inclusion:** A focus on perfection can lead to the exclusion of people who are perceived as different or "not good enough." Embracing imperfection allows us to celebrate diversity and create a more inclusive motherhood experience.
3. **Reduced competition and comparison:** When we focus on achieving perfection, it can lead to competition and comparison with others. This can create a sense of isolation and inadequacy. By accepting imperfection, we can create a more supportive and collaborative environment. When we reduce competition and comparison, our village can grow exponentially.
4. **Greater tolerance and understanding:** When we accept that imperfection is part of the human experience, we are able to be more tolerant and understanding of others' mistakes and shortcomings.

Practicing flexibility in parenting is not about giving up or settling for mediocrity. It is about accepting that we are all human and that we will all make mistakes. It is about focusing on progress, not perfection, and learning and growing from our experiences. When we embrace flexibility in parenting, we can create a more positive and fulfilling life for ourselves and for our kids.

Striving for Perfection Has a High Cost

Perfectionism has long been associated with decreased satisfaction. When we practice perfectionism, we burn out. We burn out not only in our family lives but also in our work lives. The pressure to perform becomes so great that we demonstrate increased anxiety and depression by falling into the trap of believing that perfection in motherhood can exist.

Take a moment to read through this list. Make a mental note or write down in your journal how many of the following thoughts or actions you've experienced in early motherhood.

1. You feel like a failure if something doesn't go as you planned.
2. You find yourself in the trap of comparison with other moms.
3. You believe you need to be an expert on all things child related.
4. You have rigid expectations for yourself and your kids.
5. You find yourself focusing on mistakes.
6. You worry that you'll be judged by your child's imperfections.
7. You feel anxious and stressed about day-to-day parenting decisions.
8. You feel the need to schedule every detail of your day.
9. You have a hard time delegating tasks regarding the baby to those around you.
10. You find yourself prioritizing appearance and maintaining a certain image.

If you identified with four or more of these points, we can venture to say that you could use practice at leaning into flexibility. Rest assured: If you're reading this list and nodding yes again and again, you aren't alone.

I'll say it, I'm happy to: The perfect mom doesn't exist, and the idea of a perfect mom is BS. It's an unattainable myth that's become so drilled into our idea of how we *should* parent that it impacts our ability to enjoy parenting. That shimmering image of a mom who never falters, never tires, and effortlessly juggles career, family, and PTA meetings with a perpetually radiant smile—she doesn't exist. The perfect mom that bakes Pinterest-worthy cupcakes while never being tired, touched out, or bored—she doesn't exist either. And here's the twist: This standard that we place on ourselves to be the perfect mother usually takes away from our ability to become the mother that we want to be. Yet the pressure to reach some unattainable standard of perfection in motherhood is real, and it ties directly into the notion that if you aren't the perfect mom, are you even momming in the first place?

So, if I'm not the perfect mom, am I even momming? Yes. The answer is yes. Even if you aren't the "perfect mom," you are still momming. And you're likely still momming really well. There is no such thing as a perfect mom, and you don't have to strive for it.

Before we move on to the next chapter, let's try some simple exercises that you can do right now to begin a practice of flexibility in postpartum that you can carry with you throughout your motherhood experience.

Road Map to Change Exercises

BRIEF AND PRACTICAL WAYS TO PRACTICE THOUGHTFUL FLEXIBILITY IN MOTHERHOOD

Have you had times when you felt that motherhood is a constant battle with chaos?

Let me reassure you: It's okay if things don't go as planned. It's okay if dishes sit in the sink overnight. It's okay if laundry piles up. It's okay if your partner doesn't parent the same way you do. Motherhood is an ongoing practice in surrender.

When you feel like you're not doing enough or doing well enough, I encourage you to ask yourself: What is the worst that will happen if *x* goes unattended to? And if the worst really does happen, will it matter?

The relationship between control and perfectionism is significant and multifaceted. Both perfectionism and control often stem from a desire to know or determine the outcome, our image and processes. Here are a few ideas for practicing imperfection, or what we will call newly found flexibility in our parenting.

Identify and Acknowledge What's Out of Your Control

Make a list of things that are out of your control. These little, everyday moments remind us that postpartum life is unpredictable, messy, and often comically frustrating. No amount of planning can prevent these hiccups, which is why flexibility isn't just helpful—it's essential. By recognizing these factors, you can release yourself from the stress of trying to control them. Here are a few ideas to start:

- Baby having a blowout right before leaving
- Cluster feeding at the worst times
- Unexpected spit-up on your fresh outfit
- Traffic making you late to an appointment
- Baby sleeping in the car but waking up when you get home
- The stroller meltdown in public
- Delayed doctor's appointments with a hungry baby
- Receiving a package or loud knock just as baby falls asleep

- Running out of wipes at the worst possible moment
- Technology failing during virtual check-ins or work calls

1. As you begin to notice the out-of-your-control moments in day-to-day life, also begin to make note of the way you are talking to yourself in those moments. Understanding that these situations are unavoidable can help you shift your focus from frustration to acceptance. Let's use an unexpected blowout while you're getting ready to leave the house as an example. Do you find yourself saying "I should have known better than to schedule something out of the house" or "Okay, curve ball. Let's get you changed, and let's be on our way"? Do you notice the difference? One is steeped in self-criticism, the other in flexibility.
2. Make it a daily practice: At the end of each day (or in the moment, if you can), take a minute to reflect on the unpredictable moments that threw you off course. Write them down or simply acknowledge them in your mind. Then notice how you responded. Were you self-critical, or did you allow yourself some flexibility?

If you find yourself slipping into frustration or self-blame, try reframing your inner dialogue. Instead of *I should have been more prepared*, try *That was unexpected, but I handled it.* The goal isn't to eliminate frustration entirely—it's to recognize when you're being unreasonably hard on yourself and practice shifting toward self-compassion. With time, this exercise will help you build resilience, laugh at the chaos, and remind yourself that perfection isn't the goal—adaptability is.

Shift Your Self-Talk

Self-talk is the internal dialogue we have with ourselves, shaping how we interpret experiences and respond to challenges. It can be positive and encouraging or negative and self-critical, influencing your emotions, confidence, and decision-making. In motherhood, self-talk plays a powerful role in how moms navigate stress, setbacks, and the unrealistic expectations placed on them.

This exercise works because it helps you reduce self-criticism by being honest about the things that are out of your control. You can eliminate self-blame and negative self-talk when there is traffic that you had no way of knowing would impact you. You can alleviate extra stress by acknowledging that you aren't actually able to manage every aspect of every scenario a day may present. And you can enhance your flexibility in your expectations, which will help you roll with the punches of postpartum life.

Start by catching yourself speaking negatively to yourself. Then follow these six steps. Each time you recognize self-criticism creeping in, return to this process. The more you practice, the more natural it will feel, and over time, you'll notice a shift in how you respond to challenges.

1. **Notice the negative patterns:** Pay attention to recurring thoughts that are self-critical or unrealistic, like *I'm a bad mom because my baby won't stop crying*. Simply recognizing these patterns is the first step toward changing them.
2. **Challenge the thoughts:** Ask yourself *Would I say this to a friend?* or *Is this thought based on fact or just self-judgment?* Replacing harsh self-criticism with more balanced perspectives can help shift your mindset.
3. **Reframe with self-compassion:** Replace negative thoughts with gentler, more supportive ones. Instead of *I'm failing*, try *I'm learning, and I'm doing my best*. This small shift can make a big difference in how you feel.
4. **Use affirmations that feel true:** Instead of forcing positivity, choose affirmations that resonate, like *I am enough*

just as I am or *My baby doesn't need perfect; they just need me.*

5. **Surround yourself with supportive voices:** Whether it's a trusted friend, a therapist, or an online community, hearing affirming messages from others can reinforce a more compassionate internal dialogue.
6. **Celebrate small wins:** Acknowledge what you *are* doing well, even if it seems small, like getting through a tough night or asking for help when you need it.

Shifting negative self-talk is a practice, not an overnight fix, but every time a mom replaces self-judgment with self-compassion, she takes a step toward a healthier, more empowered mindset.

Finding Calm When Everything Feels Out of Control

Remember: When something is out of your control, it isn't personal. And it's not a reflection of your value, ability, or desire. Here are some simple tactics to choose from when everything feels out of control.

1. Focus on what you can manage or control: your own reactions, how you spend your time, and who you spend your time with.
2. Delegate tasks to your support people. Less on your plate = less to manage = less stress.
3. Practice setting realistic expectations: High or unrealistic expectations can lead to frustration, feelings of inadequacy, and disappointment. Instead, set realistic and attainable goals for your day, and focus on progress rather than perfection.
4. Celebrate your mistakes: Parts of parenting are skills that we learn over time. When have you ever tried something

and it was perfect the first time? I would put my money on almost never. At least for me.

5. Change the way you talk to yourself when you've made a mistake: Instead of all-or-nothing thinking, remind yourself often that a lot of life exists in the middle and that each "mistake" is a growth opportunity in disguise.
6. Focus on what you're learning, not where you feel you're failing.
7. Find humor in the chaos: My whole parenting experience shifted when I allowed myself to laugh at the absurdity of life with a little one.
8. Let yourself laugh: Don't be afraid to laugh at the mishaps, figuring it out, the messy parts of parenting. It's not fun being the parent whose kid is melting down in public, but also, it's part of parenting. I'd rather have a laugh than beat myself up. Also, wouldn't it be amazing if we could also melt down in public when we feel like it?

Three Important Things

At the very end of each chapter, I'll note three important takeaways from each chapter. After my three, I encourage you to write down your biggest takeaways for easy reference.

1. Just because history has told you that you have to be perfect doesn't mean it's true; the myth of the perfect mom is made up. And you don't have to participate in the myth of perfection anymore. This is your permission to reject it.
2. Outdated standards are outdated for a reason. Be the rule breaker, be the warrior, and set your own new and improved standards.

3. Replace the words *imperfection*, *failing*, and *the worst* with *flexibility*. Instead of "I'm totally failing my baby," try, "I'm working on being flexible, and my baby and I will be better off for it."

What's coming next? I leave you with this question: When you think of the perfect birth, what comes to mind?

2

The Myth of the Perfect Birth

On October 5, 2017, the harvest moon, a full moon that occurs near the autumnal equinox, rose over Colorado. The harvest moon has long been a symbol of abundance, offering farmers extra light to gather their crops. (It's also a beautiful Neil Young song.) That same week, Denver witnessed an extraordinary migration of painted lady butterflies. The orange-and-black beauties, often mistaken for monarchs, swarmed the city in such numbers that someone told me they appeared on weather radars.

I was living in Colorado at the time, and I captured a video of the painted ladies fluttering in the garden at my workplace. It's the last thing saved on my phone before I became a mom: On October 6, my water broke.

I was thirty-seven weeks and two days pregnant, and according to an old wives' tale, a full moon can pull babies into the world just as it stirs the tides. And so, as if by nature's design, our son, Jack, arrived in the quiet space between a painted lady migration, a harvest moon, and the season's first snowfall. He came surrounded by beautiful forces of nature. It sounds like the perfect birth, doesn't it?

Now if I were to fill in each of the details surrounding those seventy-two hours, one might not walk away with warm and autumnal vibes. What if I told you that I pushed for four-plus hours, had a provider put their whole arm in me to rotate the baby, had an epidural fall out and put back in during deep contractions, was a puking machine, and was *hiiiiigh* as a kite when my son arrived? Would your feelings change? Or what if I shared that during my unplanned but also nonurgent C-section, I heard a provider say, "I'm seeing more blood then I'd like to," which kicked me right into *Okay, great, this is where I die; my son and I die; everyone's dying*? Thankfully, nobody was dying, we were all healthy, but at the time, while my abdomen was open and I was awake, I was convinced that everyone was not going to be okay.

Two things can be true at the same time: I became a mom during a perfect fall weekend, and parts of my birth scared me. Both are the beginning of my story as a mom. Just like there is no such thing as perfection in motherhood, there is no such thing as a perfect birth.

The beginning of any story serves as our entry point, just as our first contraction begins the process of becoming a mother. The beginning establishes the setting, introduces the characters, the mood, the meaning. The beginning also provides a foundation for our experiences and shapes the lens through which we see and internalize our own starting points. In motherhood, this beginning is pregnancy and then childbirth. And often, our birth holds the lens through which we first glimpse motherhood, a profound and intimate experience that shapes our initial steps into our new role. If that lens is clouded by fear, pain, or disappointment, it can cast a shadow over the whole experience of early motherhood.

The stories that we hold on to, the narratives we carry—they are part of our personal identities, our relationships, our views of motherhood. The stories we tell ourselves reflect our values, morals, and goals. Our understanding of pregnancy and birth is often shaped by the stories we've inherited—parental anecdotes, religious texts, historical accounts—and they become our primary reference points. These narratives, while undoubtedly meaningful, can create our own expectations around birthing and obscure the diverse realities of what happens in childbirth.

I recently asked my podcast cohost Ruby, "When you think of the perfect birth, what comes to mind?" And without hesitation, she said, "A birth at home, with no interventions. Which is crazy, because that isn't how I birthed and it's *far* from what I wanted for myself." We've been trained to think that pain means danger, blood means danger, and loud noises mean danger. Birth can be filled with all three, and all three are natural—not always a sign of danger. In my quest to understand all the myths that we hold around birthing and "a perfect birth," I started by looking at the stories I'd been told.

Growing up, I had three primary sources of information regarding pregnancy and birth:

- My own mom, who conceived easily and birthed without interventions, assisted by a midwife, in the 1980s.
- My mom's mom, who had three C-sections in the 1950s due to limitations in her own mobility. She had osteomyelitis from tuberculosis as a child and was able to achieve only minimal hip mobility.
- My dad's mom, who suffered many miscarriages between having three boys. She experienced depression and years of untreated hypothyroidism.

It wasn't until after I had given birth that I was able to understand how my view of success in birthing came to be. I realized that my perceptions were deeply influenced by these stories. But I hadn't realized that I had subconsciously absorbed the belief that a "successful" birth was one with minimal interventions and uncomplicated by medical conditions. Yet my own experience taught me that success in birth isn't defined by the absence of interventions or complications but in the well-being of the mom and baby.

If the stories you've absorbed paint a picture of an idealized and perfect birth, the reality of a challenging birth can be especially jarring. Feelings of loss, disappointment, and even failure can overshadow the joy of welcoming a new baby.

The Stories You've Been Told

What are the stories you've been told, and how did they become a marker for your own success or failure in birth? Here are a few good reflection questions to start better understanding the ways you've internalized expectations around birth.

1. How have the birth stories you've heard from friends or family shaped your expectations or fears about your own birthing experience?
2. Can you identify specific moments or conversations that influenced your perception of what constitutes a "successful" birth? If so, how did these shape your feelings during and after your pregnancy?
3. Have you felt pressured to meet certain standards or ideals around your birthing experience?
4. How might reframing your birth story—in a way that focusses on resilience, strength, and love—change how you perceive your own experience?
5. What would it mean for you to redefine success in birth on your own terms, independent of the stories or experiences of others?

Once you've taken time to reflect on these questions, the next step is to use your insights to shift your perspective and release unrealistic expectations. Here's how:

1. **Identify patterns and pressures:** Look for recurring themes in your answers. Were you told that a "good" birth means avoiding interventions? That epidurals are a sign of weakness? That C-sections mean failure? Recognizing these ingrained beliefs is the first step toward letting them go.
2. **Acknowledge your unique experience:** Every birth story is different, and comparing yours to someone else's doesn't change its value. Your birth experience is yours alone—it doesn't need to meet anyone else's definition of success.
3. **Reframe your story:** Instead of focusing on what didn't go as planned, try rewriting your birth story through a lens of resilience, strength, and love. What challenges did you overcome? How did you show up for yourself and your baby in ways that mattered?
4. **Redefine success on your own terms:** Let go of external expectations and decide what success means for *you*. Maybe it's advocating for yourself during labor, making an informed choice, or simply doing the best you could in the moment.
5. **Turn reflection into self-compassion:** When self-doubt creeps in, remind yourself that birth isn't a test you pass or fail—it's an experience. Your worth as a mother isn't defined by how your baby arrived but by the love and care you give moving forward.

By working through these steps, you create space for healing, self-acceptance, and a more compassionate view of your own story—one that honors both the challenges and the strength it took to bring your baby into the world.

Kate's Story

Kate came to see me after her second child was born. She was feeling deeply unsettled by the experience. She had always dreamed of a calm, "natural" birth—the kind of serene, effortless delivery she saw depicted in movies and on social media. When she was pregnant, she spent months preparing for this "perfect birth," reading birth plans, practicing breathing techniques, and visualizing the experience. But when the big day arrived, things didn't go as planned.

Kate's labor was long and complicated. After hours of trying to manage the pain naturally, she ended up needing an emergency C-section. When she looked back on the experience, she felt like she had failed.

"I don't understand why I feel so disappointed," she said in one of our first sessions. "I have a healthy baby, but I can't shake the feeling that I didn't give birth the 'right' way. It wasn't like what I was told it should be."

Kate had fallen victim to the myth of the perfect birth—the idea that there's one ideal way to bring a baby into the world, and anything less than that is somehow inadequate. This myth is pervasive in media and social circles, which often idealize natural births while marginalizing the many ways in which babies can be born—whether through C-sections, inductions, or medical interventions.

Her feelings of inadequacy were compounded by well-meaning but hurtful comments from others. Some friends and family expressed their surprise that she had a C-section, as if it were something to be ashamed of. "Next time, try for a natural birth," one person said, unintentionally deepening her sense of failure. And to add to her already complicated feelings about her second birth, her first birth—uncomplicated vaginal with epidural—had laid the groundwork for her wanting an intervention-free second birth.

Through our work together, Kate began to see that her experience was valid, even if it didn't match her immediate idea of what a birth should be. We talked a lot about how birth is inherently unpredictable and how unpredictability doesn't define success or failure. Kate came to realize that she could long to have had a different experience and be proud of what she accomplished at the same time. She also came to realize that the idea of a "perfect" birth was an unrealistic expectation, one that left little room for the messy, complex reality of childbirth.

By the end of our sessions, Kate had reframed her experience. She stopped viewing her birth as a failure and started embracing it as a testament to her strength and resilience. "It didn't go the way I thought it would," she said, "but I got through it, and my baby is here, and that's what matters."

Kate's journey reflected her need to break free from the myth of the perfect birth—a myth that too often leads new moms to feel like they've failed when, in fact, they've been brave and powerful in ways that transcend any preconceived notion of what childbirth "should" look like. In exploring the different narratives she had inherited regarding what makes a birth "worthy," Kate was able to detach her story from an idealized story, and it allowed her to be present instead of racked with guilt.

When we take a closer look at how we've absorbed the narratives around pregnancy and giving birth, we can scrap the idea that there is one perfect way to give birth to a baby. And when we share our own stories, we reclaim our own experiences and ascribe new meaning to the beginning of our experience in parenthood. I have had two cesarean births. I know that for many, this isn't considered "natural," but I can assure you that had I given birth at almost any other time in history, my babies and I would all have had a poor outcome. Understanding this and practicing self-compassion as well as recognizing my courage and my ability to safely bring my babies into the world has allowed me to be proud of myself as a mom and as a woman.

Giving Birth at Thirty-Two Weeks

I love how birth stories are profound narratives of transformation that unfold when a person becomes a mother. I also love how the reflections of our births change with time; we settle into them and they become part of the bigger story instead of the whole story.

I'd love to share the birth story of my daughter with you.

In May 2020, right after the world had shut down and we were beginning to understand the scope of what a global pandemic might be, I gave birth to a little baby girl, affectionately named Ruby, at thirty-two weeks. And her birth was empowering as hell.

On May 20th, I was woken up by contractions. I had lost my mucus plug, the jellylike plug that forms in the cervix during pregnancy and seals the cervical canal, creating a barrier that protects the uterus and aids in fending off infection. As a woman approaches labor, the cervix begins to thin, sometimes causing the mucus plug to be expelled. Mine was expelled, without hesitation, as if to say *Here you go, sis. Get ready for the ride of your life.*

I took a quick shower, and I drove myself to the hospital before work—visitors weren't allowed, and masks were required. When I arrived at the hospital, I was sent to triage, where the baby and I were monitored for an hour. After that hour, a midwife came into the room to tell me that, yes, I was in fact having contractions, but they weren't regular, and contractions aren't abnormal to experience at thirty-two weeks in a second pregnancy. I was sent home with instructions to stay hydrated and rest.

On the ride home from the hospital, I called my mom, hysterically crying. I told her I really didn't want to have a baby at thirty-two weeks during a pandemic. I didn't want my baby to go to the NICU, I wasn't prepared to leave work yet, we hadn't even set up her bassinet, I didn't want to leave the hospital without my baby girl. I was crying about all of the factors that I had zero control over, and I wasn't ready to let go of my perceived control just yet. If motherhood is anything, it's a daily lesson in surrender. Ruby taught me that. She also showed me that I was meant to be her mother and grow alongside our little preemie lady. She's taught me so much.

I got home, headed to my office, and worked the whole day. By four thirty PM I was having regular contractions—they were five to seven minutes apart. I called my ob-gyn and told her I was pretty sure I was in labor, so she asked me to come back to the hospital. I asked her what would happen if I went into active labor at thirty-two weeks. She told me they don't do anything to stop the labor at thirty-two weeks, as the outcomes are generally positive. I grabbed my purse, gave my husband and little two-and-a-half-year-old son hugs, and headed to the hospital. Again, no visitors, masks required.

I drove myself to the hospital, parked the car, stepped out, closed the door . . . and my water broke. Standing in the middle of the hospital parking lot, alone and in labor eight weeks early at the beginning of a global pandemic.

I walked up to triage; I told them I thought my water had broken and that I was having regular contractions. They roomed me and swabbed my vagina, where they were able to confirm that my water had broken. This was it, I knew this was it. I come from a long line of strong women who do what they want and aren't afraid to break the rules. My daughter was going to do just that.

I was waiting alone for a little while. I FaceTimed my mom and my sister. If you've ever been in a highly intense, high-stakes, big-emotions situation, you know the focus and courage that takes over. This urgency was a call to my strongest self: *You are in labor, your baby is going to be born early, and you are completely capable of meeting this moment.*

My focus narrowed. I asked the questions, got the answers, and kept my baby safe. An OB came in, and she gave me the plan: They were going to do everything possible to keep me pregnant through thirty-four weeks. I was going to get some type of shot in my leg to help with the baby's lungs, and I would be transferred to a labor-and-delivery room for monitoring. I could invite my husband to come stay at the hospital with me.

Labor and delivery during the early days of the pandemic felt dystopian. The nurse swabbed me for COVID, and I swear she touched my brain; I had never experienced anything like it.

After several hours of monitoring, I was moved into a regular hospital room—at the end of the hallway where they kept a row full of moms in situations similar to mine, the "can't go home, but it isn't time yet" moms-to-be. I was told the original plan, with a few new additions—they were going to start me on IV antibiotics to avoid infection, and they would be checking on me periodically.

By the next morning, I was having regular contractions. I could still hold a conversation and walk myself to the bathroom, but I was in pain, with waves of contractions that took my breath away, and I wanted some pain meds. The hospital shifts had changed, and the new team of ob-gyns came in in the morning to introduce themselves and monitor any progress. They checked to see how dilated I was, how I was feeling, and gather any additional updates.

I told them I was in labor; I told them I was in pain; I told them I wanted pain interventions and that if I was in active labor, I would like to birth my baby. I let the doctors be doctors, and I let myself be the mom, the expert on my own body and the number-one advocate for our baby.

We agreed that they would finish their rounds and recheck to see how dilated I was when they returned. We agreed to reassess and make a new plan in a few hours. They returned; I was eight centimeters dilated and knew that I was going to be having my second C-section. And so off to the operating room we went.

A motto or mantra in my own life that I come back to often was incredibly helpful in this moment: *The outcome is already determined; I just have to figure out how to get through the process without melting down.* (Or with only brief meltdowns that I could work through, because, let's not forget, feelings are what make us human, and we aren't supposed to respond like computers.)

Baby girl was coming; the outcome was already determined. My job was to not panic.

If you've had surgery or a previous cesarean, you know that the operating room is very cold, very clean, and not meant to have too much personality. I was joined by my husband, two female anesthesiologists, two female obstetricians, one female OB fellow, several female nurses, several female NICU nurses, and a female medical assistant. And at 12:33 PM, my daughter was brought into the world by a team of talented, kind, smart, and amazing female providers. During a global pandemic. Eight weeks before her due date.

Note: Our daughter still runs the show. That is all.

The NICU staff will generally tell the caregivers of premature babies to expect that they'll be in the hospital until their original due date. Insurance had cleared me to stay in the hospital for five nights, and at the end of the five nights, I would be allowed into the NICU only once per day. I could stay for as long as I wanted but was only able to enter the building once per day. On the third morning of my hospital stay—after my husband had gone home and my mother-in-law had arrived—one of the ob-gyns who had delivered Ruby stopped by my hospital room to let me know that she herself had been born at thirty-two weeks and that my daughter was going to go on to do great things.

Over the years, I have heard hundreds of birth stories. I've heard every variety of how women have become mothers: at home with a midwife, in the hospital in a tub, low intervention, high intervention, alone, with a roomful of people, surrogacy, etc. I've worked with moms who, by medical standards, had very uneventful births, yet the moms held trauma around the experience. And I've worked with women who've had what some would consider harrowing births and weren't fazed by the experience.

In therapy I regularly ask expectant parents, "What are your hopes for your birth?" I would say 98 percent of first-time expectant parents have the same goal: to labor at home as long as possible, to have limited intervention in the hospital, and to birth vaginally. Never have I heard a new mom tell me her goal was to have a C-section. And C-section moms are quick to explain or rationalize away why their pregnancy ended in a surgical procedure instead of stitches in their lady parts. And the thing I remind moms of, as often as I can (this may be the soapbox I die on), is that every birth is a birth. You can't fail. You didn't fail. No matter how your baby came out.

The dictionary definition of birth is "the emergence of a baby or other young from the body of its mother; the state of life as a physically separate being." The definition of birth isn't about how the baby came out; it's the fact that the baby came out. It's the act, not the process.

This doesn't mean that you won't have strong feelings about your own story; it means that regardless of how your baby made its way earthside, your story is valuable and precious. Every birth is beautiful, and you get to be proud of your story and proud of the worthiness of your hard work. Always. When it comes to birth, there is no comparison, there is no failure, there is only you, your strength, and your accomplishment.

What Type of Birth Do You Imagine as Perfect?

Have you ever considered what ideas you've held as the perfect birth, either before giving birth or in retrospect? And if your birth didn't go as planned, how did this change your perception of your own abilities in motherhood? Many moms I've met tell the stories of their births with great pride—or a whole lot of explanation when it didn't go as they had hoped. If you've wrestled with the meaning of your own birth stories, I'll leave you with these few questions I regularly encourage moms to think about to explore their own biases.

1. What specific details or outcomes do you associate with the perfect birth?
2. What would ruin your idea of the perfect birth?
3. How do you think meeting your ideal, perfect birth would impact your postpartum experience?
4. If your birth was disappointing, how does that impact how well you perceive you're doing in motherhood?
5. How does a birth plan contribute to having a perfect birth?

These questions are meant to help you reflect on the sources and standards that have influenced your expectations, which can reveal underlying pressures or ideals you haven't considered before.

While I was pregnant with Jack, I was handed a birth plan form by a nurse and asked to fill it out. I had zero idea what it was and zero idea how to fill it out. I didn't have a birth plan. I thought that my water would break, I would go to the hospital, and I would have the baby. That was my plan. I hadn't realized how narrow my own knowledge of birth was until I was handed that plan, which I am pretty sure I never filled out. Remember, I come from a long line of strong-willed ladies who do what they want. It's in our DNA. Looking back now, however many years after giving birth, I can see how the stories I had inherited about birth played out in my own two birthing experiences.

In the vein of my mom's story, I worked with midwives, assuming that would be the most "natural" option. In the vein of my grandma's story, I had no opinions on cesarean birth. And in the vein of my Nona's story, my hormones were all within normal range, and I had never experienced depression, so I wasn't worried about those factors. I also have hypothyroidism and was monitored by a serious but thoughtful endocrinologist throughout both of my pregnancies.

Before I became immersed in the world of early motherhood, I sort of knew the business of birth but didn't fully understand the variety of ways that the 130 million babies born each year come into the world—130 million stories of birth waiting to be told, 130 million moms with a new badge of honor.

What About a Birth Plan?

As a therapist who works primarily with expectant and new parents, I am often asked which birthing plan I like best. While I see the value in making a plan, I've also sat with many moms while they process their disappointment after their birth has gone differently than they wished.

For the moms who like a plan (totally understand; I too am one of those moms), these are my top tips:

1. Make sure you like your provider.
2. If you can't be vulnerable in front of someone, they shouldn't be part of your birth.
3. Choose several birthing preferences—stay home as long as possible, epidural upon request, the people you would like to be there—and throw any formal plan to the wind.

Please remember, this is your birth too. You may not be the expert on the birthing process, but you are the expert on your own body and the limits of what you're comfortable with. Whether you've completed a full and detailed birth plan or you intend to wing it, remember that your voice matters.

Understanding the Stories We've Absorbed

I love history, and for me to understand our stories around birth, it's important for me to see the whole picture, the backstory, the setting, the mood, the circumstances. And I must say, researching birth trends has allowed me to move from suspicion of the birthing industry to gratitude that I gave birth during this time in history. And still, for many, the idea of giving birth at home or a birthing center, with limited interventions, remains the gold standard. How did this become the collective narrative around what makes a successful birth?

For centuries, birthing was commonly an event that took place in the community, with midwives and other women assisting, rather than a noted medical event as it is today. With the development of medical technologies, birth moved from a traditionally women-led event to a monitored event taking place in a hospital. This shift is called medicalization, the concept of non-urgent events becoming medical events treated by specifically trained professionals. The medicalization of motherhood took place largely when birth practices moved from home to hospitals. And naturally, this development created a shift in the way women were treated during pregnancy and after delivery.

This shift from community birthing to hospital birthing had natural consequences, like most things. Some positive, some not so positive. The medicalization of birth led to a change in autonomy for many birth mothers by opening their support circles to strangers (doctors) and systems that they were not stakeholders in (hospitals). Policies and procedures created by medical professionals became what defined the "right and wrong" way to birth. And then, through this medical lens, a mother's success began to be measured by an external agent as opposed to a midwife or a woman in her community. If she got birth "wrong," as determined by a medical professional, motherhood was off to a start that wasn't defined or created by the mother.

While birthing in medical settings has been beneficial in many ways—reducing maternal and infant mortality, offering pain relief options, and providing emergency interventions—it has also contributed to the idea that there is a right or wrong way to give birth. This pressure can leave women feeling like they've somehow failed.

Imagine the 1500s, a time when pregnancy was an experience fraught with uncertainty. Women, understanding the risks of labor and delivery, often prepared their wills as soon as they learned they were pregnant, ensuring their affairs were in order should they not survive childbirth. In the 1500s childbirth was predominantly a female affair. Women in the community who were skilled with generational knowledge in assisting labor were the primary caregivers during pregnancy and birth.

As we rolled into the 1600s, the role of male physicians began to emerge, mostly in more complicated deliveries. This shift reflected a growing interest in anatomy and the continued development of surgical tools—these are the earliest signs of the medicalization of the birthing process. Among the new tools introduced were forceps. Forceps offered a new way to assist in difficult births; however, they had their risks as well. (In researching this, I've now read more stories about the early use of forceps and heard far more forceps horror stories than I'd ever like to know.)

In 1765, Pennsylvania Hospital recorded the first hospital birth in the US when a baby girl was born to Martha Robinson, noted as a young and poor new mother. In 1793, the first lying-in (maternity) department at Pennsylvania Hospital was developed and officially opened on May 20, 1803; the first admission, though, had been on March 30, and the first birth—of a female child—on April 27. At this time, the majority of births were still taking place at home and in the community and hospitals were mainly utilized by the poorer classes of society.

The first recorded use of chloroform in childbirth was by Dr. James Young Simpson, a Scottish obstetrician, in 1847. He pioneered the use of chloroform as an anesthetic during labor, but it was Queen Victoria's highly publicized birth experience in 1853 that brought the practice into the mainstream. Her use of anesthesia led to a surge in its popularity among upper-class women. This marks two crucial advances in medicine: women's pain being acknowledged as significant and the introduction of pain management options during labor and delivery.

By the early 1900s, a combination of scopolamine and morphine, commonly known as twilight sleep, became a popular method of pain management during childbirth. This method was an induced state of amnesia and sedation for the birthing person. The combination of these two medications effectively erased the memory of labor pains. Basically, birthing parents were "eternal sunshined" out of remembering their labor-and-delivery process. The effects of twilight sleep included hallucinations, respiratory issues in the newborn, and an actual lack of pain relief for mothers in labor. By the 1960's, the adverse effects of twilight sleep were becoming more evident in medical communities and harder for medical professionals to ignore.

The 1920s saw another big shift as hospital births became the norm in many Western countries, particularly the United States. This movement advocated more of an interventionist approach to childbirth—hospitals provided a more sterile and controlled environment, which reduced the risk of infections and complications. The 1920s also saw a rise in the routine use of forceps, episiotomies, and anesthesia, which one could argue reflected the growing confidence in medical technology as a means of managing birth.

And, of course, when the pendulum swings one way, it will naturally swing the other way. In this case, it swung under the influence of Dr. Grantly Dick-Reed's 1942 book *Childbirth Without Fear. Childbirth Without Fear* challenged the newly popularized medical approach to childbirth, advocating a more "natural" approach. Dick-Read believed that pain in childbirth was due to women's fear, and he suggested the importance of education, relaxation, and emotional support to reduce fear and thus reduce pain.

And, up until this point, have any of these birthing experts been women? No. That's a resounding no. With only a brief mention of the role of midwives and supportive women in the community, it seems that as soon as birth moved from communities to hospitals, care shifted away from communal support—or women-led care—and toward isolation and medicalization.

Let's move on to the 1970s, another era that highlights tremendous change in birthing practices. Birthing moved away from the heavily medicalized model while embracing a more holistic, family-centered approach that acknowledged birth not just as a medical event but a deeply personal experience as well. The 70s saw the popularization of epidurals, the inclusion of fathers in the delivery room, and a broader cultural recognition of women's autonomy. *Finally* there was a focus on choosing pain management options that aligned with women's individual needs and values.

From the early 2000s until today, we have seen a significant rise in the rate of cesarean sections, accounting for approximately one-third of all deliveries by the end of the first decade of the century. This rise was attributed to various factors, including increased maternal age, medical concerns, fear of lawsuits, and changing attitudes toward surgical interventions. Today, women have a wider array of birthing options than at any other time in history. The focus has shifted to reflect a growing emphasis on personalized care and informed decision-making.

Birthing trends come and go, which to me signifies that from the start, there was never one right or wrong way to give birth. More recently it feels like the medical methods used to help bring a baby into the world are slowly shifting to focus on empowering women to make the choices that are best for them and their mental health. Birthing options today are vast, and outside of medically emergent cases, we can still see significant differences in birthing experiences and maternal preferences, also highlighting a shift in autonomy and ownership for the birthing parent.

The modern landscape of childbirth is a testament to how far we've come in recognizing that every birth is unique. Just as the standards and practices have changed over time, so too has the understanding that the perfect birth isn't defined by the absence of pain or interventions but by the safety and well-being of both the mom and baby. In this way, the narrative of childbirth continues to evolve, moving away from rigid expectations and rules and toward a more inclusive view that honors the diverse experiences of all mothers.

And yet there is still work to be done. Despite the advances in birthing practices and increased emphasis on personalized care, significant challenges remain, particularly in the United States. The US has the highest maternal mortality rate among developed nations—a statistic that is both alarming and indicative of systemic issues within our insurance and health care systems. According to the Centers for Disease Control and Prevention (CDC), about seven hundred women die each year in the United States because of pregnancy or delivery complications. Even more concerning is the stark racial disparity: Black women are three to four times more likely to die from pregnancy-related causes then white women. In my years of practice, I have never heard a white woman tell me they are scared to walk into a hospital; I have, however, heard many women of color share the sentiment that if they go into the hospital, they won't come out alive.

And these disparities are not solely about mortality. Many women experience severe maternal morbidity, which includes life-threatening complications such as hemorrhage, preeclampsia, and sepsis during and after childbirth. The CDC reports that for every woman who dies from pregnancy-related causes, there are approximately seventy women who experience a life-threatening complication during childbirth.

Of course, the reasons for these disparities are complex and multilayered. Implicit bias in health care, lack of access to quality health care, and socioeconomic disparities all contribute to the maternal health crisis. Studies have shown that Black women are often not listened to by health care providers and as a result may receive substandard care. Women who lack proper health insurance are less likely to seek perinatal care. Women who live in rural areas are less likely to seek or have access to perinatal care. Lack of accessible care can lead to delayed prenatal care, which can increase the risk of complications during pregnancy and childbirth.

While birthing outcomes have improved over the years, these statistics underscore the need for continued efforts to ensure that all women, regardless of race or location, have access to safe and effective perinatal care. Addressing these disparities requires a multifaceted approach, including policy changes, increased support for maternal health programs, and a commitment to addressing the underlying social determinants of health. The narrative of childbirth must continue to evolve, not just in terms of medical advancements but in ensuring that every woman can experience a safe and healthy birth. As we reflect on the historical evolution of childbirth and the societal shifts that have shaped our understanding of it, it's clear that childbirth, both in its medicalization and in its deeply personal nature, is not a one-size-fits-all experience. The narratives we've inherited about what a "perfect" birth should look like often set us up for unrealistic expectations, leaving little room for the reality of how different each of our births look.

Processing your birth experience is an essential step in reclaiming your own narrative, especially in a culture that has long dictated what a "successful" birth should look like. The history of childbirth shows us that standards and practices have continuously shifted, often shaped by societal expectations rather than the needs of birthing parents. These shifting ideals—whether promoting unmedicated birth as the gold standard or pushing for highly medicalized interventions—have left many women feeling like they either met or failed some unspoken test of motherhood. But birth is not a pass-or-fail experience; it is a deeply individual journey shaped by countless factors, many of which are out of our control. Instead of measuring your birth against rigid expectations, the key to healing lies in processing your experience on your own terms. By acknowledging the realities of your birth, untangling the pressures and messages you've internalized, and reframing your story through a lens of strength and resilience, you can move forward with greater self-compassion and a more empowered perspective on your journey into motherhood.

Road Map to Change: Let's Process Your Birth

To move past popularized standards and start honoring our individual experiences, a perfect place to start is by processing our own birth stories with honesty and self-compassion. While I know this can be super hard, reflecting on our birth experiences allows us not to see them through the lens of how they "should have gone" but instead to appreciate, or at the very least accept, them for what they are. In doing so, we allow ourselves the space to hold both joy and disappointment, healing and growth. And then we get to rewrite the beginning of our mothering stories.

If your birth experience didn't unfold as you envisioned it, it's important to acknowledge and move through whatever strong feelings or emotions you are having surrounding your labor and delivery. Whether your birth was a minor deviation from your hopes or a significant departure, understanding and addressing its impact can help set you on the right path to managing your well-being as a new mom.

Taking time to process your own birth story is important for several reasons:

1. **Physical healing:** The postpartum period is a time for your body to recover from the physical demands of pregnancy and childbirth. Taking time to rest and heal before diving into the emotional processing of your birth story allows you to approach the experience from a place of physical wellness. This physical recovery helps you to avoid overwhelming your system while you work through intense emotions.
2. **Emotional clarity:** Birth is a profound, life-changing event, and immediately after, emotions can be raw, heightened, and overwhelming. Allowing yourself time gives you the space to reflect and gain emotional clarity so you're not making judgments or decisions in the heat of the moment. This time allows you to process the overwhelming range of emotions—joy, fear, frustration, or even disappointment—in a more measured way.
3. **Perspective:** Birth experiences can be complex, filled with unexpected twists and turns. With time, your perspective may shift as you gain new insights. You might see things in a new light as you process your emotions, understand what you've learned, and accept the reality of what happened. This added time can help you integrate the experience, making it easier to identify areas of satisfaction or regret and begin to make peace with it.
4. **Bonding with your baby:** The early postpartum period is crucial for bonding with your newborn. Spending the first few weeks focusing on bonding, breastfeeding, and adjusting to new routines can help you settle into motherhood before diving into your birth narrative. This allows you to

process your birth story in a way that doesn't feel rushed or influenced by exhaustion or overwhelming emotions.

5. **Reduced postpartum stress:** The birth experience can bring up a mix of intense emotions—especially if things didn't go as planned. Rushing to process it too soon can add to postpartum stress and anxiety. Giving yourself time allows you to process the experience in a way that's more manageable and less likely to negatively affect your mental health.
6. **Healing and empowerment:** Taking the time to process your birth story can be empowering. It allows you to examine your experience and understand what was within your control and what was not. It helps you regain a sense of agency, whether you feel satisfied with the outcome or need to work through parts that were traumatic. This process of self-reflection can be healing and supportive of emotional growth.

Taking time to process your birth story will help you approach it with emotional clarity, physical recovery, and a deeper understanding, which will foster healing and empowerment as you navigate the postpartum experience.

When you process your birth, you experience powerful benefits, including the ability to:

1. accept your experience and find closure,
2. reduce trauma's grip,
3. allow yourself to deepen the growing bond you have with your baby,
4. prepare for potential future pregnancies,
5. reduce stress and anxiety,
6. enhance your physical recovery,
7. strengthen your boundaries and communication,
8. foster empathy for yourself,

9. embark on a journey of growth, and
10. leave a legacy of love without fear.

Depending on how your birthing experience went, you might feel ready to start processing your birth right now, or you might not. The following exercise is meant to help support you, so move forward in processing your birth in the way that feels safest for you right now. It is meant to span an eight-week period, but that is merely a suggestion. Please feel free to complete it within your own timeline.

As you begin exploring your feelings around your birth, here are some key points to keep in mind:

1. Every woman's birth experience is unique, and there's no right or wrong way to feel or process it.
2. Be patient with yourself and allow yourself time to heal physically and emotionally.
3. Don't hesitate to seek support from loved ones, professionals, or other new moms. You're not alone in this journey.

Road Map to Change Exercise

THE EIGHT-WEEK GUIDE TO PROCESSING BIRTH

Weeks 1–2: Focusing on Rest and Recovery

1. **Physical healing:** Prioritize rest, sleep when the baby sleeps, eat nutritious meals, and stay hydrated. Allow your body to recover physically from labor and delivery. Follow any postpartum care instructions from your health care provider.

2. **Emotional adjustment:** Acknowledge your feelings, whether joy, exhaustion, or a mix of emotions. It's normal to feel overwhelmed. Share your thoughts with your partner, family, friends, or a therapist.
3. **Bonding with baby:** Spend time cuddling, feeding, and caring for your newborn. Skin-to-skin contact fosters a deep connection.

Weeks 3–4: Reflect and Reconnect

1. **Journaling:** Write about your birth experience, including your feelings, thoughts, and any details you remember. This can be a therapeutic way to process your experience. This is a perfect time to start working through the guided journal prompts titled "Questions and Considerations" (page 54) to process your birth.
2. **Talking to your partner:** Discuss your birth experience together, sharing your perspectives and feelings. This can strengthen your bond and provide mutual support.
3. **Seeking support groups:** Join a new-moms group or online forum to connect with other women who recently gave birth. Sharing experiences and offering support can be incredibly beneficial.

Weeks 5–8: Integrate and Move Forward

1. **Professional help (if needed):** If you're experiencing postpartum depression or anxiety, don't hesitate to seek help from a therapist or counselor specializing in maternal mental health. (See Chapter 9 for more about postpartum depression or anxiety.)
2. **Celebrating your strength:** Recognize the incredible feat of bringing a new life into the world. Celebrate your resilience and the love you have for your child.

3. **Creating a birth story:** Consider creating a tangible birth story in the form of a scrapbook, photo album, or even a short video. This can be a treasured keepsake for you and your child.

Questions and Considerations for Processing Your Birth

Whether you are doing this work on your own or working with peers, a doula, or a therapist, here is a list of journaling prompts. These prompts aim to guide you through reflecting on your birth experience with compassion and clarity, allowing for healing, understanding, and integration of the experience into your identity as a parent.

Reflecting on Your Birth Experience

- What are the first thoughts that come to mind when you think about your birth?
- What moments during labor or delivery stand out to you the most?
- Was there anything unexpected that happened during your birth? How did you feel in those moments?
- How did you feel about your body during labor and birth? Were there any surprises or challenges?

Emotions and Feelings

- How did you feel in the hours and days after your birth? Did your emotions shift over time?
- Did you experience any feelings of fear, joy, frustration, or disappointment during birth? How did you cope with them?
- Did you feel supported by your birthing team (partner, doctor, midwife, doula)? Why or why not?
- How did you feel about the choices you made during labor (pain relief, interventions, etc.)?

Your Support System

- What role did your partner or support person play during your birth? How did they make you feel?
- Was there anyone you wish had been there for you during birth, or someone you're grateful was there?
- How did your caregiver (midwife, doctor, nurse) contribute to your birth experience? Did they support your preferences?

Unexpected Events or Disappointments

- Was there a part of your birth plan that didn't go as expected? How did you feel about that change?
- Were there any decisions made during your birth that were difficult for you to accept?
- How do you feel about the overall outcome of your birth? Were there things you feel at peace with, or are there aspects you still feel conflicted about?

Physical Experience

- What was your experience with pain during labor? How did you manage it?
- How did your body feel during labor and delivery? Were there parts of the process that were physically difficult?
- How are you feeling physically now, after having gone through birth? Do you notice any lingering effects or changes in your body?

Postpartum Healing

- How are you feeling emotionally and physically in the days and weeks after birth?
- Are there any things you wish you had known or prepared for in the postpartum period?

- How has your relationship with your baby evolved since birth? What moments of connection stand out?
- How have your relationships with others (partner, family, friends) changed since your birth?

Your Birth Story and Identity

- How has your birth story shaped your identity as a mother?
- What lessons have you learned about yourself through your birth experience?
- What are you most proud of when you think about your birth experience?
- How do you want to share your birth story with others, and what message do you want to communicate about it?

Regrets, Resentments, and Healing

- Are there any parts of your birth that you feel regretful or resentful about? What would it take for you to heal from those feelings?
- How can you practice self-compassion as you reflect on your birth experience?
- Is there anything you need to forgive yourself for in relation to your birth experience?

Looking Forward

- How can you use your birth experience to inform your future decisions or plans (whether for future births, parenting, etc.)?
- What do you wish you could tell other women about birth after going through your own experience?
- What advice would you give your past self during your pregnancy now that you've gone through childbirth?

The way you feel about your birth today will likely change over time. I encourage you to revisit these prompts and revisit your birth story from time to time; it will teach you new things about yourself with each revisit. A few things to keep in mind moving forward, or in planning for subsequent labor and deliveries:

1. **Self-care:** Continue to prioritize your physical and emotional well-being. Make time for activities you enjoy, even if it's just a few minutes each day.
2. **Open communication:** Talk openly with your partner, family, and friends about how you're feeling. Don't hesitate to ask for help when you need it.
3. **Embrace the journey:** Motherhood is a continuous journey of learning and growth. Embrace the challenges and cherish the joys along the way.

The myth of the perfect birth isn't just a story; it's a standard we have been taught to measure ourselves against, often without even realizing it. Whether your birth experience was empowering, challenging, ordinary, or full of unexpected turns, it was yours—and it deserves to be honored for what it was, not measured against an impossible ideal.

The truth is, there is no singular way to define a "perfect" birth. Birth is unpredictable and deeply personal. It can be joyful, painful, transformative, and even traumatic—all at once. The goal isn't perfection but resilience, connection, and finding our own way through. When we allow ourselves to release the grip of this myth, we make room for something far more powerful: the ability to embrace our birth stories in all of their complexities. We give ourselves permission to grieve what didn't go as planned, celebrate what did, and find strength in the fact that we did the best we could with the information and resources we had available at the time.

The myth of the perfect birth is a distraction from the reality that all birth stories are valid and meaningful. By rejecting this stupid myth, we can focus on what truly matters: safe, supported, and individualized care and the knowledge that perfection isn't required to bring a baby into the world—or be proud of ourselves as parents.

Your story is part of you; it's not all of you, and it's not a measure of your worth. It's not about perfection; it's about the love, courage, and humanity you bring to motherhood every single day.

Three Important Things

1. There is actually no such thing as a perfect birth, and if you're disappointed with how your birth went, it's time to process it.
2. Thank goodness none of us had to birth in the 1500s.
3. As polarizing as the birthing industry feels, we are pretty lucky to be living in a time where we at least have some autonomy over our experiences.

What's coming next? I urge you to answer this question: Which came first, bonding with your baby or caretaking with no feedback?

3

The Myth of the Perfect Way to Feed Your Baby

When you first held your baby, what were the thoughts that crossed your mind about feeding? Did you feel sure of yourself, or did you wonder if you were doing it right? For many of us, the path to feeding our babies isn't always straightforward. It's filled with questions, moments of doubt, and plenty of what-ifs shaped by what we've been told, how we were raised, and what we see around us. From the very start, feeding becomes part of a bigger story—a story that carries both personal meaning and the weight of expectations from others.

In the debate over what the "right way to feed a baby" is, we often miss one very important part of the conversation: feeding your baby is so much more than choosing between breastfeeding, formula, or both. It's an ongoing journey that's connected to your relationship with your baby, your sense of self, and the world around you. Along the way, there are reflections: What's working? What feels good? What's been harder than you expected? And maybe, most importantly, how do you balance your personal feelings with the pressures you feel from others?

In this chapter, I'm hoping we can all take a pause and reflect on our own experiences in feeding our babies, whether we're at the very beginning of figuring it out or close to the finish line. We'll think about the emotions that come with feeding, how outside expectations have shaped our choices, and how we can embrace our experience—just as it is. Wherever you are in this process, my hope for you is that you feel empowered to honor your journey and trust that whatever path you take is the right one for you and your baby.

The Great Dilemma: Breastfeeding Versus Formula

When I go to visit friends who have just had a baby, I stick to a specific script. I walk in and assess the scene: Is there laundry that needs to be done, dishes that need to be cleaned, counters that need to be wiped, or a dog that needs to be walked? Does the new mom need a nap, a shower, a break from holding the baby? I know that asking for help can be really hard, and sometimes new moms don't want even their most trusted friends to handle the baby. So I enter, I assess, and then I offer a helping hand.

One day I walked into my friend's house, took the dog out, and came back asking if they had a to-do list I could tackle. This specific friend just wanted company, and I was more than happy to offer a listening ear. "I don't want to breastfeed; I don't want to pump," she shared. "It's too much touching, it's too much noise, it's too time-consuming. I don't like doing it. And I'm too embarrassed to tell anyone. I'm making milk and feel like I should want to be nursing, but I don't want to nurse," she said.

"Then stop," I said. "You don't need to explain. If it isn't working for you, it isn't working, and that's okay."

There are a million reasons a mom will breastfeed and a million reasons a mom will choose formula. One mom's best way to feed is going to be another mom's nightmare. Breastfeeding, bottle feeding, formula feeding, feeding on demand, feeding on a schedule—these are all very personal choices. The myth that there is one "right" way to feed your baby has become a divisive force among mothers, fueling guilt, shame, and an inaccurate sense of inadequacy. The mommy wars over feeding choices are fueled by such strong identities on both sides, and as a therapist, it's awful to watch. New moms have enough going on; they don't need additional layers of self-doubt thrown in.

It's important that mothers know they have permission to feed their baby in the way that is best for them, even when the choice can feel very difficult, for so many reasons. The pressure to conform to societal expectations, the well-meaning advice from friends and family, and the pervasive myths about "the right way" can create an overwhelming sense of uncertainty. Mothers often feel that their decision is a reflection of their parenting abilities, and that can make the process feel even more emotionally charged.

In addition to external pressures, there are also deeply personal factors at play. Some mothers may feel a sense of guilt if they can't breastfeed or have to supplement with formula. Others may feel sadness or frustration if breastfeeding doesn't come as naturally or easily as they had hoped. The fear of not providing the "best" for their baby can cast a shadow over every feeding choice, even though each method can provide nourishment, love, and connection.

It's also important to recognize the physical and emotional toll that these decisions can take. The fatigue of late-night feedings, managing milk supply, and navigating a baby's changing needs can leave mothers feeling drained, both physically and mentally. The right decision can be an act of self-care in itself, allowing moms to prioritize their own well-being alongside their baby's needs.

Ultimately, the most important thing is that mothers are empowered to make the choice that aligns with their values, their health, and their unique family dynamic. There is no one "correct" way to feed a baby—what matters is that the method chosen fosters a connection between mother and child, allows the mother to feel supported and confident, and promotes a nurturing environment for both.

Modern moms haven't been trained to tune in to their own wants and needs—at least, not without guilt or second-guessing. From the moment we enter motherhood, we're flooded with messages about what's "best" for our babies, often at the expense of our own well-being.

For so many moms, the process of feeding a baby becomes an exercise in self-sacrifice rather than self-awareness. The idea that what's best for the baby must always come first can overshadow the truth that a thriving baby needs a thriving mother. And yet, because so few of us have been encouraged to listen to our own inner voice, it can feel radical—almost selfish—to make choices that consider our needs alongside our baby's.

But what if we shifted the conversation? What if instead of focusing on the *right* way to feed a baby, we focused on what allows a mother to feel nourished, capable, and confident in her choices? What if we gave mothers permission to listen to their instincts, trust their bodies, and make feeding decisions based on *both* their baby's well-being and their own?

Feeding a baby isn't just about calories and nutrients—it's about connection, sustainability, and finding a rhythm that allows both mom and baby to thrive. When we learn to recognize and honor our own needs, we free ourselves from the impossible standard of perfection and step into something far more powerful: the ability to mother in a way that feels right for *us*.

Making a Feeding Decision When There Are a Lot of Opinions

Breast is best. Fed is best. Exclusive breastfeeding. Combo feeding. Formula feeding. Pumping. Donor milk. Each option comes with its own set of expectations, rules, and—more often than not—judgment from others. Instead of being encouraged to ask questions—*What works best for me? What does my body need? What will allow me to show up as the healthiest, most present version of myself?*—we are handed external scripts that tell us what we *should* do. We weigh our choices not just against our personal realities but against cultural ideals that don't always take into account our emotional, physical, or financial circumstances.

Feeding an infant is far more than a practical decision about nutrition. It's deeply intertwined with emotions, expectations, personal identities, and family dynamics. As a therapist, I've witnessed how making a choice about feeding can shape parents' emotional experiences during the early months of parenthood. By understanding the emotional considerations that accompany our feeding choices, parents can approach feeding with more clarity, self-compassion, and confidence. Beyond advice from medical providers, navigating the social expectations can be the hardest part for many new moms. For many new moms, it is assumed that they are going to breastfeed on demand, with the assumption that this is the only and right option for all moms. But this just isn't the case.

After our son was born, a lactation consultant encouraged me to go to a lactation group at the hospital where I gave birth. I had chosen to breastfeed, and Jack and I were getting the hang of it, but I was in a stage where I didn't know how much milk he was drinking, so I liked the idea of going to a weighted feed, which is where your baby is weighed, you nurse them, and then they are weighed again to get a ballpark idea of how many ounces they've eaten. The lactation consultant who referred me to the group reassured me that it was a great group of new moms, feeding in all different ways, and many had continued to come for the social aspect even if they no longer needed lactation support. I forced myself to go. I didn't want to go, but I did, if only for the sake of getting used to leaving the house with my baby, nursing in public, and most importantly, allowing myself to be vulnerable.

While the benefits of breastfeeding are well documented, this immense social pressure around it creates a lot of stress for a lot of new parents. Mothers may feel that their ability to breastfeed defines their worth as a parent, woman, mom, caretaker, and postpartum person. And, for bottle-feeding parents, the stigma around formula feeding can manifest in subtle or overt judgements. I've heard many moms share that they've received comments about nursing being the "natural" choice by friends, family, and strangers, who question why they would choose any other method. And then we face the social judgment around feeding in public. Nursing in public, no. Giving a bottle in public, no. A crying baby in public, no. A postpartum mom just trying to figure it out, no, society has told us they don't want to see that either.

Biases about infant feeding don't just exist on the surface; they run deep, shaping how mothers perceive their own choices before they've even made them. From the moment a woman becomes pregnant, she is inundated with messaging about what's *best* for her baby—messages that often come wrapped in judgment and moral undertones rather than true support.

For many, the expectation of exclusive breastfeeding is framed as a moral imperative rather than a personal or logistical decision. Hospitals encourage it, lactation consultants reinforce it, and well-meaning family members question any deviation from it. On the other side, formula feeding—despite being a completely safe and viable option—is often met with side-eye glances, unsolicited opinions, or undertones of pity, as if a mother must have "failed" in some way to end up there. These biases don't just come from society at large; they exist within us too.

Why Parents Might Choose Formula

There are a number of very valid reasons a new parent wouldn't nurse their baby. Here are just a few:

1. Inability to change or discontinue medications: Mental health medications and medications necessary for certain health conditions that cannot be discontinued and are not compatible with nursing.

2. Low supply: Certain conditions make breastfeeding physically difficult or impossible.
3. Previous surgeries or injuries: A history of breast surgeries can impact milk production.
4. Birth of multiples: Producing enough milk or managing breastfeeding for twins, triplets, etc., can be difficult.
5. Maternal illness: Conditions like HIV, untreated TB, and cancer requiring treatment are incompatible with breastfeeding.
6. Infectious diseases: In certain situations, breastfeeding can pose a risk of transmitting infections.
7. Postpartum complications: Conditions like severe postpartum hemorrhage or emergency surgeries can delay or inhibit breastfeeding.
8. History of trauma or abuse: Past trauma, particularly sexual trauma, can makes breastfeeding emotionally complicated, triggering, or dissociative.
9. Returning to work: Workplace accommodations for pumping are sometimes lacking, and time constraints can come into play.
10. Cultural norms or stigma: Community beliefs or cultural practices may discourage breastfeeding.
11. Shared caregiving: A partner, family member, or caregiver may share feeding responsibilities.
12. Lack of support: Inadequate access to lactation consultants, breastfeeding education, or community support can discourage breastfeeding.
13. Lack of desire: Sometimes mothers simply don't feel a desire to breastfeed. It's as simple as that.

14. Financial barriers: Limited resources may make necessary breastfeeding supplies (pump, milk storage options) unaffordable.
15. Medical conditions in the baby: Prematurity, tongue-tie, cleft palate, etc., can preclude breastfeeding.
16. Unable to latch: The infant may not latch effectively or prefer bottle feeding.
17. Adoption or surrogacy: The biological mother may not be available to breastfeed.
18. Allergies or sensitivities: Babies may react negatively to something in the mother's milk.

Most mothers don't enter parenthood as blank slates. We absorb stories from our own upbringing, our cultural background, our peer groups, and even our health care providers. If we grew up with a mother who breastfed effortlessly, we might assume we should be able to do the same. If we were formula fed ourselves, we may carry unconscious beliefs about its sufficiency. If we've been part of certain parenting communities, we may have internalized strong stances about what "good" mothers do—even when those beliefs don't align with our actual lived experience.

These biases don't just dictate how we feed our babies; they dictate *how we feel about how we feed our babies*. A mom who chooses formula may feel the need to overexplain, to justify her decision in the face of unsolicited opinions. A mom who exclusively breastfeeds may feel pressure to keep going even when her body is depleted. A mom who combo feeds may feel like she's failing to commit to either "side." And yet, when we strip away the cultural conditioning and personal biases, the reality remains the same: Every mother is making the best decision she can with the resources, information, and circumstances she has.

By recognizing our own internalized biases, we can begin to approach feeding decisions with more clarity and self-compassion. Instead of feeling trapped by expectations, we can ask ourselves *What do I truly need? What allows me to be the best version of myself for my baby?* When we make space for these questions, we create room for a feeding journey that is not just about sustenance but about confidence, connection, and a deep trust in our own ability to mother in a way that feels right for us.

When we create an environment where new moms can't win, we all lose. When we aren't encouraging postpartum moms to explore different feeding options and to explore what is best for them, we are failing them. Imagine what would happen if we created a loving environment for new moms to heal, feed in a way that works for them and felt supported with no guilt for the choice they make? What would happen if we approached feeding our babies with neutrality as opposed to hostility? I bet new moms would feel much more supported, and freer to parent authentically.

Breast Milk and Its Alternatives in History

I'm not here to be a cheerleader for either side of the feeding debate, breast milk or formula; I'm here to be your cheerleader in whatever method you choose. There are benefits to both, and there are many reasons you might choose one feeding method over the other. And any variety works if it works for you. I'm not going to tell you what a doctor thinks you should do—please consult them directly with any medical questions. Instead, we're going to look at the cultural landscape and the trends in how we feed our babies. We're going to validate the choice you already made, and we're going to put this mommy war to rest.

Ancient Bottles and Animal Milk

The study titled "Milk of Ruminants in Ceramic Baby Bottles From Prehistoric Child Graves," published in *Nature* in 2019, revealed that bottle feeding is far from a modern invention, as prehistoric babies were fed animal milk using small ceramic pots.

Researchers analyzed small, spouted ceramic vessels excavated from infant graves in Bavaria dating between 450 and 1200 BC. Chemical analysis of the lipid residues inside these vessels revealed the presence of ruminant milk, indicating that prehistoric communities used these "baby bottles" to feed animal milk to infants. This discovery provides direct evidence of supplementary feeding practices in prehistoric human groups. Bottle feeding isn't new! Supplementing with alternatives to breast milk isn't new!

Throughout history, breastfeeding has been essential for infant survival. And, for most of history, there was also an absence of alternatives. For mothers who were unable to nurse, wet nurses—women who breastfed others' children—became a solution, ensuring a continuity of care. Wet nursing began as early as 2000 BC, with "lactation failure" being included in the earliest medical encyclopedia, the Papyrus Ebers, which came from Egypt in 1550 BC. The prescription for a mom with an inability to produce enough milk for her infant was as follows:

> To get a supply of milk in a woman's breast for suckling a child: warm the bones of a sword fish in oil and rub her back with it. Or: let the woman sit cross-legged and eat fragrant bread of soused durra, while rubbing the parts with a poppy plant. (Wikes, 1953)

To any mom reading this who has dealt with low supply, please be comforted by the fact that we are parenting in an age where we have alternate options for infant nutrition. I, personally, would be pissed if I was trying to nurse and someone was rubbing me with poppy plants. It's also worth noting how low milk supply has been recorded in history for at least the last four thousand years. *Repeat after me, please: Low supply is not a moral failing!*

Eventually, breastfeeding as a necessity grew in value and became an essential piece of what is considered maternal duty. Still, history tells stories of wealthier families employing wet nurses to feed their young.

It was common for wet nurses to be employed by aristocratic and royal families, as breastfeeding was seen as incompatible with the lifestyle of elite women, who often prioritized maintaining their social demands or physical appearances over the role of feeding their babies. In royal courts, wet nurses' proximity to royal children could offer them some influence within the residence.

In ancient Egypt, royal mothers often delegated nursing duties to wet nurses, who were in turn honored with statues or inscriptions. Wet nursing offered a perfect alternative for mothers who were unable or unwilling to nurse their babies. Wet nursing has a whole dark history of its own that I would encourage you to read about if it interests you. You can take a deep dive into the world of breast milk as a commodity, but for the sake of supporting you in the decisions you make around feeding, we're going to fast-forward to the invention of formula.

The invention and popularization of formulas in the late nineteenth and early twentieth centuries dramatically transformed the role of wet nurses. In the mid-nineteenth century, scientists began creating early forms of infant formula as an alternative to breast milk. Justus von Leibig, a German chemist, developed one of the first widely marketed infant foods in 1867, made of cow's milk, wheat flour, and potassium bicarbonate. Companies aggressively marketed formula as modern and scientific, emphasizing its convenience and positioning it as a safer, more hygienic alternative to wet nurses. These campaigns targeted middle- and upper-class families, who were, as we've learned, the primary employers of wet nurses.

Leibig's Soluble Infant Food was the first commercial baby food in the United States, selling in grocery stores for $1 a bottle in 1869. This would be equivalent to $63.82 today. In the 1870s, Nestlé's Infant Food, made with malt, cow's milk, sugar, and wheat flour, became available in the US, selling for $0.50 a bottle. Nestlé's formula was diluted with water, requiring no cow's milk to prepare, and thus was the first complete artificial formula available in the United States.

As public health campaigns began to emphasize the importance of sterilization and sanitation, formula feeding was promoted as a more controlled and less risky way to feed infants, particularly in urban areas where access to clean water and hygienic conditions for nursing might otherwise have been limited.

The rise of formula marked a turning point in infant feeding practices. Formulas provided increased convenience and accessibility and reflected broader social changes, including industrialization, urbanization, and a shift toward the importance of medical advice. But as we've learned, nothing ever remains the same, and the development of feeding technologies met its match when the pendulum swung the other way back toward breastfeeding as the superior option for feeding.

The 1970s in the US and Europe saw a resurgence of breastfeeding. After decades of decline due to the rise of commercial formula feeding, the 1970s produced a reaction to women's liberation movements of the 1960s that emphasized bodily autonomy and a more "natural" form of parenting. Breastfeeding was marketed again, and this way as a way for women to reclaim their bodies from medical institutions and corporations.

Advances in scientific research in the 1960s and 1970s began to highlight the immunological and nutritional properties of breast milk, and research suggested that breastfeeding reduced infant mortality, infections, and chronic diseases. Organizations like the World Health Organization and the American Academy of Pediatrics began advocating breastfeeding as the optimal feeding method.

How Infant Formula Has Changed From 1870 to Today

In the 1870s, infant feeding alternatives were often homemade, using diluted cow's milk with added sugar or cream. These mixtures were imprecise and lacked nutrients, unfortunately leading to high infant mortality rates.

From 1900 to 1940, advances in pasteurization and sterilization made formulas safer by reducing contamination. Manufacturers also began to modify formulas to mimic breast milk's fat content, introducing cream-based formulas. By the 1920s and 1930s, formulas were fortified with essential vitamins and minerals, such as vitamin D to prevent rickets.

After 1940, scientists began altering cow's milk proteins to make the formula easier for babies to digest, with the 1950s seeing the introduction of iron fortification to combat infant anemia. The 1960s brought soy-based formulas for babies with lactose intolerance or cow's milk protein allergies. This is the time when companies like Similac and Enfamil became household names, marketing heavily to new mothers.

The 1980 Infant Formula Act in the US established minimum nutritional standards and safety regulations for infant formula. Companies began researching human breast milk composition and reformulating products to include whey protein, essential fatty acids, and better carbohydrate sources.

In the 1990s, formulas began including omega-3 and omega-6 fatty acids, which are critical for brain function and development. Modern formulas also include ingredients to support gut health and immunity, mimicking the benefits of breastfeeding. Options now exist for preterm infants, babies with allergies, and babies with specific medical needs. And reflecting consumer demand, many brands now offer organic and non-GMO formulas. Looking at the development of infant formula over time shows a scientific and historical account of trial and error with cutting-edge science, leading to a safe and nourishing alternative for families who need or choose it.

By the 1980s, research on the benefits of breastfeeding began to gain traction, and organizations like La Leche League, which had been advocating breastfeeding since the 1950s, saw renewed support. The World Health Organization (WHO) and UNICEF launched the International Code of Marketing of Breast-Milk Substitutes in 1981 to curb formula companies' misleading advertising practices, especially in developing nations where formula use was linked to higher infant mortality due to lack of clean water.

In the 1990s, the Baby-Friendly Hospital Initiative (BFHI) was introduced to encourage hospitals to support breastfeeding through practices like immediate skin-to-skin contact and rooming-in. While breastfeeding rates started to rise, formula was still widely used, and many women faced structural barriers—such as short or nonexistent maternity leave—that made exclusive breastfeeding difficult.

By the early 2000s, breastfeeding advocacy was at an all-time high. The American Academy of Pediatrics (AAP) issued strong recommendations for exclusive breastfeeding for six months and continued breastfeeding for at least a year. Celebrities and influencers began publicly normalizing breastfeeding, and social media allowed for widespread lactation education and advocacy.

However, this era also saw the rise of *breastfeeding pressure* and *mommy wars*—heated debates over what constituted "good" mothering. Formula feeding, while still common, became increasingly stigmatized in certain parenting circles. Many mothers who struggled with breastfeeding felt guilt and shame, and the phrase "Breast is best" became both a rallying cry and a source of pressure. Meanwhile, structural barriers, such as inadequate parental leave policies and lack of workplace accommodations for pumping, made exclusive breastfeeding an unrealistic goal for many mothers, exacerbating feelings of failure.

The current cultural landscape surrounding breastfeeding and formula feeding is loud and shaped by many different voices—medical, social, economic—as well as personal preference. The World Health Organization and the American Academy of Pediatrics currently recommend exclusive breastfeeding for the first six months of life, with continued breastfeeding alongside solid foods until at least one year or beyond. *And* formula feeding is recognized as a nutritionally adequate and safe alternative. Modern formulas are scientifically designed to closely mimic the nutritional profile of breast milk, providing essential nutrients for infant growth and development.

What's crucial here is to acknowledge the changing cultural attitudes around what is expected from new moms. My mom, born in 1954, was formula fed; everyone was using formula at that time. My mom, being a product of the 1970s, felt comfortable nursing until she was done and then supplementing with formula. My sister and I were breastfed and then formula fed. My kids, born in 2017 and 2020, were breastfed, bottle fed, and given cow's milk at twelve months. I started supplementing my breast milk with formula for my first baby when he was eleven months old. We all did our best, which is what I think most moms aim for—to get our babies fed to the best of our ability.

The pressure to choose the "right" method often begins during pregnancy, and then in the hospital, and it can be detrimental to the new moms who are struggling with it. Family members, friends, and even strangers contribute to this pressure with unsolicited advice and critiques. Similar to the C-section moms who feel the need to explain away their birthing choices, formula-feeding moms find themselves experiencing moral judgments and an external scrutiny that leaves them feeling as though their feeding choices are public property and open to debate.

Even without external judgments, mothers often wrestle with internal conflicts. Those who struggle to breastfeed may feel they are failing at a fundamental aspect of motherhood, while those who choose formula from the outset may feel defensive about their decision. This internalized guilt can lead to feeling anxious and sad and add to a diminished sense of confidence in parenting. The myth that there is only one right way to feed your baby places an enormous emotional burden on mothers, leaving many feeling caught in a no-win situation where any deviation from the ideal is perceived as a failure. And this is where I'd love to say *Who cares what anyone thinks?*—and I do say this in therapy—but the truth is that an unsupported mom becomes a mom who thinks she's failing.

Maggie's Story

Maggie came to see me for the first time when she was a few weeks postpartum. She knew she was going to be returning to work, she was excited and confident in that decision, and she wanted a little extra support as she was preparing to make her transition. Shortly before returning to work, Maggie and I ended up in a session discussing breastfeeding, formula feeding, and everything in between. "I thought I would love it," she said, shaking her head. "I really did."

"Breastfeeding?" I asked.

She nodded. "It was supposed to be this beautiful bonding experience. I read all the books, followed all the lactation consultants on Instagram, joined the support groups. But in reality? It was awful. It hurt, he was constantly hungry, and I felt like I never had a second to myself." She ran a hand through her hair. "I thought it would get better, but it didn't. And now my maternity leave is ending, and I just—" She exhaled sharply. "I could not picture myself hooked up to a pump in the middle of my workday."

I nodded, letting the weight of her words settle. "That's a big shift. What was it like making that decision?"

Maggie hesitated, then let out a small laugh. "Honestly? I felt guilty, like I was failing some invisible test. But also—relieved. Like, really relieved. I told myself I'd try pumping at work, just to see. But the first day I sat in that tiny lactation room, exhausted and stressed, and I thought . . . why am I doing this to myself? I wasn't even sure who I was trying to prove something to."

"And what happened when you decided to stop?" I asked.

She smiled—an easy, genuine smile. "I went out and bought formula that same night. And you know what? I've never looked back. I don't have to time my meetings around pumping, I don't feel that constant pressure to keep up my supply, and best of all, I enjoy feeding my baby now. Like, really enjoy it. I hold him, I look at him, and I feel present. I thought stopping would feel like a loss, but it actually gave me so much more."

I smiled. "Sounds like you made a choice that honored both you and your baby."

Maggie nodded. "Yeah. I thought I had to love breastfeeding. I thought if I didn't, something was wrong with me. But the truth is, what I really needed was to love how I was feeding my baby. And I do. I really do."

Maggie wasn't failing; she was being honest and being true to herself and what worked for her. She let herself be unbothered by any external expectations and tapped into what was working for her, for her mental health and physical health, and in turn, everyone wins! Lack of desire is a valid reason that doesn't reflect her value as a mom.

Social Inequities in Feeding/Economic Factors

We have already seen the role of wet nursing and social inequities, but we have yet to explore feeding choices that are also shaped by systemic inequities. Access to lactation consultants, breast pumps, and leave varies widely, which leaves many mothers without the resources to make feasible choices.

The economics of infant feeding are significant and often overlooked in broader conversations. Breastfeeding is portrayed as free, but this disregards the hidden costs. Many breastfeeding mothers need pumps, storage bags, nipple creams, specialized bras—all of which can add up quickly. And then there is the time spent breastfeeding or pumping—often *many* hours each day. All of these can hinder a mother's ability to return to work or manage other responsibilities.

For formula-feeding families, the financial burden can be even greater. Formula is expensive, and the cost increases as babies grow and consume more. Low-income families may struggle to afford formulas. The economic realities add layers of stress for many mothers already grappling with the pressures of feeding decisions.

Marginalized mothers—from communities of color, immigrant populations, or low-income backgrounds—face their own challenges in feeding their babies. Additionally, studies have shown that low-income mothers are less likely to receive access to high-quality lactation support or affordable formula options, while immigrant mothers often encounter larger barriers and cultural stigmas that hinder feeding choices. These systemic inequities create tangible barriers to both breastfeeding and formula feeding, exacerbating disparities in maternal and infant health outcomes.

Mothers in marginalized communities may also face greater stigma, no matter their feeding choice. A Black mother using formula might be judged as uninformed, while a Latina mother breastfeeding in public could be criticized for immodesty. These intersecting prejudices magnify their effects and the isolation that many new moms already feel.

To address these intersecting prejudices, systemic changes such as increased cultural competency training for health care providers and the expansion of community-based support networks that validate diverse feeding choices would benefit many new parents. Policies that ensure equitable access to lactation consultants, affordable formula, and proper workplace accommodations for all mothers can also help to mitigate these challenges.

Formula-feeding mothers can be made to feel as though they've taken the "easy way out" or aren't providing the best for their child.

This stigma can foster a culture of silence and shame. Mothers may avoid seeking help for fear of being judged. This isolation can exacerbate feelings of inadequacy and undermine their confidence as parents. To combat this, we must move toward a more inclusive and compassionate view of infant feeding, one that celebrates the diversity of maternal experiences rather than policing them.

The narrative around feeding babies has long been dominated by the idea of "the best way"—an underlying standard that pits mothers against each other. It's time to ditch that whole thing. This singular focus on "best" implies a one-sized-fits-all solution that ignores the complexity of our individual circumstances, values, and needs. What it does is foster unnecessary guilt and shame if we don't meet this pretend standard of perfect.

Jess's Story

Jess and I met for the first time when her baby girl was four weeks old. In our fifteen-minute consultation, she had shared with me that she was having a hard time feeding her baby, she had seen a handful of other professionals, and she thought it was time to process through what she had expected and what her reality looked like. She walked into my office, sat down, and got straight into it.

"I just didn't think it would be this hard," she began.

Jess had always imagined that she would birth her baby, the baby would be handed to her, and they would latch. She had attended breastfeeding classes, acquired highly rated nursing pillows, bought every variety of lactation cookie, and rented a hospital-grade pump when she was leaving the hospital. And, from the moment her daughter was born, nursing hadn't gone as planned.

Despite help from multiple lactation consultants, she was in pain, latching wasn't happening, and her baby grew frustrated at the breast. Jess had been triple feeding—attempting to nurse, pumping, and then bottle feeding—and she knew this wasn't sustainable. The baby didn't have any mouth ties; she'd gotten the okay from PT and OT that everything was looking good. At her most recent appointment with the pediatrician, Jess had been provided education on formula and told she could supplement if she would like to.

"I feel like I've already failed my daughter," she admitted.

She met me at a crossroads: She could exclusively pump, or she could switch to formula. She shared that neither of these options was ideal, and she was having a hard time accepting that feeding her baby was going to look different from what she had thought. "I wanted to nurse her. I wanted that connection. Now I feel like I'm failing at the most basic thing a mom should be doing," she said, looking at me, waiting for a reply.

I thought for a moment and then said, "I'm sorry this hasn't gone how you had anticipated. I know that can be really hard.

First, we're going to explore why you feel like a failure, and then we'll work through the rest. There is no road map for navigating guilt and disappointment when our expectations don't match the reality of what's working. But we'll get you to a place where you are able to zoom out."

We talked about all the effort she had already put into feeding her baby—she needed to understand that she wasn't failing. The outcome wasn't what she wanted, but her actions demonstrated incredible efforts, instinct, and hard work. Over the span of a few weeks, we worked on her mindset and reframing her feeding options as acts of love and care. Whether she chose to exclusively pump or formula feed, she was ensuring that her baby was nourished, growing, and happy. She practiced self-compassion, becoming able to remind herself of her own worth and validating that her value as a mother wasn't tied to her ability to breastfeed.

We also explored the grief she felt about letting go of breastfeeding. Jess needed space to honor that loss without minimizing it or rushing to "fix" it. And most importantly, we focused on the relationship she was building with her daughter beyond feeding. Jess started to focus on the connection that was already growing between them, and these small moments reminded Jess that she was already creating a secure, loving bond.

During the earliest days of meeting, Jess was insistent on pumping and then bottle feeding. After a few months, she shared with me that she had decided to switch to formula. She felt that pumping was taking bonding time away from her and her daughter, and she just wanted to be able to make a bottle and focus on the bond they share while bottle feeding. Feeding her baby wasn't what she had anticipated, but she was leaning into loving what worked for them. She learned to let go of the unrealistic expectations she'd carried into motherhood and embrace a feeding choice that worked for her family. Most importantly, she realized that being the type of mom she wanted to be wasn't about meeting any external standard but about building an honest and authentic relationship with her baby.

And with that, we moved on. Jess was happy with where she had landed and was glad she had chosen a route that felt the best for her and allowed her to have a little more peace and a lot more confidence in her ability to trust herself in her role as a mom.

How We Can Change the Narrative

For too long, the conversation around infant feeding has been shaped by rigid expectations, ranking certain choices as superior and leaving mothers to navigate unnecessary guilt and judgment. But what if we shifted the focus from what's "best" to what's "best for you"? What if we created a world where feeding decisions weren't loaded with shame or pressure but were instead met with support, resources, and respect? This change isn't just the responsibility of individual parents—it's a cultural and systemic shift that requires action from health care providers, corporations, policymakers, and communities.

Here's what we can do on a larger scale:

1. **Shift the language.** Terms like *failure to breastfeed* carry deeply ingrained biases and reinforce harmful hierarchies. Instead, we must adopt neutral and supportive language that acknowledges all feeding methods as valid. Health care providers, lactation consultants, and parenting resources should lead the way in reframing these conversations.
2. **Ensure access to evidence-based, noncoercive feeding information.** Misinformation and pressure—whether pushing exclusive breastfeeding at all costs or encouraging formula without proper guidance—only fuel uncertainty and guilt. All parents deserve comprehensive, unbiased education about their feeding options so they can make choices that align with their lives, health, and needs.

3. **Normalize feeding diversity.** Every mother deserves to feel confident feeding her baby, whether that means breastfeeding in public, bottle feeding with formula, using donor milk, or some combination of these. We need a cultural shift that rejects stigma and embraces the full spectrum of feeding choices.
4. **Recognize that responsive caregiving—not just milk—is what truly nourishes a baby.** Love, connection, and attunement are the foundations of emotional security. No parent should be made to feel that the way they feed their child dictates their worth or ability to bond.
5. **Advocate workplace policies that support all feeding choices.** Paid parental leave, adequate lactation spaces, and flexible work schedules should be standard, not privileges. At the same time, workplaces should recognize that not every mother wants or is able to pump—and that should be respected without question.

But change doesn't just come from institutions. It comes from us too. So what can you do in your own community?

1. **Change the conversation.** The next time a friend, family member, or fellow mom talks about feeding struggles, lead with support, not assumptions. Ask *What's working for you?* instead of *Are you breastfeeding?*
2. **Speak up against judgment.** If you hear someone shaming a mother—whether for nursing in public or for using formula—push back. A simple "Actually, there's no one right way to feed a baby" can go a long way in dismantling stigma.
3. **Share your story.** Whether it's with a close friend, on social media, or in a local parenting group, telling your feeding journey without shame helps normalize all experiences and lets other moms know they're not alone.

4. **Support new mothers with real help.** Instead of questioning their feeding choices, ask what they need. Bring them a meal, hold the baby while they rest, or simply listen. This is how we build a culture of true support.

When we move away from the idea of one "right" way to feed a baby and embrace a "best for you" approach, we empower mothers to trust themselves. We create space for families to make choices without fear of judgment or exclusion. And, ultimately, we build a world where feeding a baby isn't about proving something—it's about love, connection, and the freedom to choose what truly works.

When we allow ourselves to embrace a "best for you" approach, we empower mothers to make choices rooted in their own needs and intuition. By doing this, we can begin to free ourselves and others from external pressures and celebrate the beauty of personalized parenting.

Shifting the conversation from "best" to "best for you" is about reclaiming autonomy and celebrating the diversity in each of our experiences. It acknowledges that every mother, baby, and family is unique. Breastfeeding might feel empowering and fulfilling for one mom while another is thriving because formula exists. Neither choice is inherently superior; the best method is the one that supports you and your baby's health and well-being.

Road Map to Change: Learning to Listen to Your Mama Choices as Valid

How we feed our babies doesn't have to be a source of guilt or division among mothers. What truly matters is learning to listen to ourselves and nurturing our children in a way that works for us and our unique circumstances. Feeding is a deeply personal decision influenced by a web as dynamic as you are. You are allowed to let go of unrealistic pressures and harmful judgments. Instead of striving for perfection or conformity, you can focus on listen to your body, tuning in to your baby's needs, and embracing whatever feeding experience reflects your values and realities. There is no one "right" way, or one universal road map, and that's okay—because feeding your baby with love and intention, no matter the method, is what matters the most.

Becoming a mom can often feel like stepping into a world filled with noise—advice from experts, opinions from family, unsolicited comments from strangers. With all this external pressure, it's easy to second-guess yourself and wonder if you're making the "right" choices. But the truth is, the "right" choice isn't something you'll likely find outside of yourself—it's learning to lean in to our own maternal instincts. Learning to listen to your own voice and trust your decisions is a skill, and like any skill, it can be strengthened over time.

Road Map to Change Exercises

REFLECTION EXERCISE: LISTENING TO YOUR INNER VOICE

Take a moment to reflect on the decisions you've made as a mom so far. How many of them were driven by others' opinions versus what felt right for you? How can you begin to recenter your choices around your needs and values moving forward? Write down any moments where you felt particularly confident in your choices, even if they were small.

Now that we've practiced listening to your inner voice, let's pivot a bit to building confidence in our decision-making as new moms.

DEVELOPING SELF-CONFIDENCE IN YOUR DECISION-MAKING

Confidence in early motherhood won't happen overnight. It takes time and practice to get to a place where you can trust your instincts, let alone have complete faith in them. As new moms, it's common to outsource our concerns to perceived experts. But it's just as important that we learn to listen to ourselves.

Trusting yourself, even when you don't have concrete answers or all the facts, is part of the process. Think of making choices as a new mom as being like picking out dressing at the grocery store—there are eight thousand choices, and it can feel overwhelming. But usually we know what we want if we listen to ourselves carefully. Learning to trust your instincts can feel like walking a tightrope, but remember: You are the one who knows your baby the best, and you are the one who knows yourself best. Instead of scrolling through social media for answers, you can use these steps to narrow down your options and find what works for you.

1. **Get quiet, tune in:** To hear your inner voice, you need moments of quiet. Take time to pause—whether during a quiet moment with your baby or while in the middle of a task. Tune in to how you feel about a decision before seeking external input.
2. **Identify your hard No's:** Learning what you don't want is just as valuable as understanding what you do want. Identifying your nonnegotiables helps clarify your decision-making process and makes it easier to trust yourself. For example, you might not be comfortable with your baby being in the car with nonfamily members. You are allowed to identify this as a hard *no*.
3. **Envision your preferred outcome:** What would be your ideal result, even if it's not perfectly achievable right now? Setting a goal helps you focus on what truly matters to

you and narrows your options to those that feel aligned with your values. These scenarios come up a lot with deciding on child care. Start at the end, and work your way backward when exploring your options.

4. **Narrow down your options:** If you had to pick just two or three choices, which would you prefer? Allow yourself to cancel everything else out. This step eliminates overwhelm and makes space for what truly feels right for you.
5. **Practice self-compassion:** As you make decisions, remember to be kind to yourself. Second-guessing is normal, but practicing self-compassion helps ease the pressure of getting everything "perfect." If you feel confident in your decision, trust that it's enough.

By practicing these steps, you'll begin to build a strong foundation of confidence in your decisions, whether they're about feeding, sleep training (or not training), or any other aspect of your early postpartum experience. While the newness of welcoming a baby makes every decision feel hugely critical, remember that if you are safe and your baby is safe, you have time to find the solutions that work best for you, your values, and your family. You are the expert!

Remember that there is no single "right" way to feed your baby. Whether you choose to breastfeed or bottle-feed or a combination of both, as long as it's working for you and your baby, it's the right choice. When you are able to make decisions that align with what you really want, you are working to create a more fulfilling and sustainable experience for both you and your baby.

You don't need to conform to anyone else's idea of "the right way." Instead, you're allowed to trust your body, your baby, and your own wisdom. As you learn to tune out the noise and lean into your own confidence, you'll find that the choices you make—whether big or small—are the ones that matter most, because they reflect your unique postpartum experience.

Three Important Things

1. One of the most important things you can do is learn to believe in yourself and the choices you are making as a new mom.
2. You are allowed to gather information and make the best and most informed decision without taking into account what others might want for you.
3. You are going to face a lot of judgment in motherhood. Stand strong in what you know is right for you, and don't make yourself small to make others feel important.

And what's next? I'll leave you with this question: Did you feel bonded to your baby immediately?

4

The Myth of the Perfectly Innate Mother

Out of the thousands of pictures I've taken since becoming a mom, one stands out as the most relatable to most postpartum parents. It's a photo of my son, Jack, on his one-month birthday. He's dressed in a carefully chosen outfit, lying on a beautiful rug in his nursery. But instead of the serene image I had imagined, Jack is hysterically crying. Behind the camera, I was crying too, overwhelmed, exhausted, and alone at home with my little baby. I remember looking at his delicious little face, and as if talking to an adult, I said, "Please be nice to me; I have no idea what I'm doing."

I, rightfully so, had no idea what I was doing . . . yet. I had been a mom for exactly thirty days. My desire to get the one-month milestone picture was in total opposition to the reality of what the moment looked like: a tired and hungry baby, in pants for the first time, alongside a tired and hungry first-time mom, also in (sweat)pants for the first time. That moment and that photo taught me crucial lessons in motherhood, like:

1. **Picture-perfect only exists online.** Which I knew but didn't, like, *know* know. I was so excited to be capturing this milestone. We had made it to one month, through little sleep, learning how to nurse, and lots of anxiety. I was

proud of us! And, also, I had convinced myself that we could caption the perfect picture to demonstrate how great we were doing. But that isn't how life with a newborn actually works. They don't care about picture-perfect.

2. **Postpartum is the greatest equalizer.** And it's okay to not know what you're doing. Even experts on attachment, therapists, psychologists, child development experts, and physicians must figure out how to care for their new baby, just like the rest of us. My mom told me once, "Babies aren't the complicated ones, adults are the complicated ones, and we make caring for a baby more complicated than it needs to be. I feel sorry for modern moms; they have so much pressure on them to do everything perfectly."
3. **We can fight change, or we can surrender.** I had an idea of how I thought our photo shoot would go, and my son had a different idea. He forced me out of an idealized version of the one-month celebration straight into the reality of caregiving. I had to learn to surrender what I thought would be cute for the photo albums to meet the reality of the moment. He had to poop. And I had to help. That day, I learned how to surrender. And in that surrender is the space where I became a mom.
4. **Knowing how to care for a baby isn't innate.** We all have to learn how to do it. Bonding is one thing, attachment is another thing, maternal instinct is another, and the learned skills of parenthood are the umbrella over the rest of it.

This is one of those persistent myths about early motherhood, which we'll call the myth of intuitive caregiving: the idea that parents, and mothers in particular, are born knowing how to care for an infant and raise them into adulthood. As if giving birth unlocks ancient wisdom encoded in our DNA that tells us exactly how to soothe a cry, interpret needs, and become a fairy-like mother goddess overnight. This myth of intuitive caregiving has been passed down from generation to generation, reinforced by cultural narratives and used to reinforce the belief that if you can't immediately care for a baby without any guidance, you are doing something wrong. And this just isn't true. This is the myth of intuitive caregiving, suggesting that if a mom has to learn, practice, or is even struggling in their new role, she is somehow failing.

The reality is that caregiving is a skill—a set of behaviors and responses that we learn through experience, observation, and trial and error—and is not always intuitive. Many aspects of parenting—feeding, soothing, understanding your baby's cues—are skills that require learning, practice, and time. Learning is a naturally imperfect process. Unlearning the idea that we should know everything about being a parent the instant we become one is a powerful step in reclaiming motherhood as an experience unique to each of us, and one where we are allowed to falter.

While maternal instinct and bonding are real to some degree, they are often romanticized in ways that exclude the messiness and individuality of real-life parenting. When my son was a few months old, I signed up for a mommy-and-me music class. Why? Actually, I have no idea. I think my stress over getting out of the house with a newborn in winter should have been reason enough to stay home, but I knew a few moms in the class and figured I should socialize.

"I don't feel like I know what I'm doing. When am I supposed to know what I'm doing?" another new mom asked me. We were sitting on the floor of this noisy music class, our newborns lying on the floor facing us.

"I mean, I don't know. Does anyone know? I surely have no idea what I'm doing yet. I feel like we've been lied to?" I responded.

At that point, I had been a practicing therapist for years, well versed in the theories of newborn and infant care. I knew the clinical definitions of bonding, attachment, maternal instinct, and other popular parenting ideals, but as a new mom myself, what was supposed to happen, when it should happen, and how it should happen all felt blurry and vague.

In my mind, caring for my baby was supposed to be like a light switch that turned on when my baby was born. I figured that I would give birth, see the baby, hold the baby, love the baby, and then, like magic, I'd know exactly how to care for him. But realistically, how would I have known how to wash a baby's neck creases? I'd never done it before. Hell, I hadn't even known babies would have folds that needed to be cleaned. In these moments, I learned that so much of early motherhood is about learned skill and not innate ability magically unlocked.

While parts of early parenting are biological, much of it isn't biological at all. This idea that we're supposed to be instantly bonded to our babies is a falsehood that I've seen rack new moms with guilt. The belief that we're supposed to feel an immediate, overwhelming connection to our babies is a cultural fiction, not a universal truth. And yet it's a fiction that has seeped into our collective psyche so deeply that when the instant bond doesn't happen, it leaves many mothers drowning in guilt and self-doubt.

Is an Instant Bond Between Mother and Baby a Real Thing?

Learned maternal behaviors and the ever-elusive attachment, bonding, and maternal instinct aren't the same thing. Here's a breakdown of these different concepts.

- **Learned maternal behaviors** are the skills we develop through experience, observation, or support from others.

These include things like soothing techniques, diaper changes, and knowing when our baby is overtired. Nobody is born knowing how to burp a baby, and we don't know until we learn.

- **Bonding** is the emotional connection you feel with your baby. It's personal and can happen in moments, or it can take time to develop.
- **Attachment** is a process; it's about building a secure relationship between you and your baby, over time, through consistent care and responsiveness. It's not instant but grows as you and your baby get to know each other. We'll talk more about attachment in Chapter 5.
- **Maternal instinct** is another way of saying "learned maternal behaviors." While certain instincts—like responding to a crying baby—are biologically driven and part of our survival instincts, much of what we call instinct is learned or developed through trial and error.

Bonding with our baby doesn't always feel automatic. The myth that new moms are just supposed to know what to do and how to care for a new baby is one of the most common concerns that brings moms to my office. Mothers may feel like they're failing because they haven't learned to decipher their baby's cues or they struggle to soothe their child. Even seemingly simple tasks, like finding the right bottle, can become a source of stress when the pressure to be a perfect caregiver lingers loudly in the background. I've met with many new moms who are riddled with guilt and sunk into the belief that they should know exactly what to do as soon as they're handed their baby.

Parenting is a constant work in progress, one that unfolds over time, filled with imperfect moments, trial and error, and a lot of learning along the way. The bond between a mother and child isn't forged in an instant, nor is it dictated by some innate knowledge of what to do. It's built in everyday experiences.

Does motherhood come naturally for some? Yes.

But not always, and not for every new parent.

While the biological basis for bonding and nurturing exists, the concept of a universal, unwavering "maternal instinct" isn't as simple as we've come to believe. The idea of a fixed, automatic set of instincts in moms is far more nuanced than *See baby, love baby, raise baby, and partake in all caregiving.*

When we meet our baby for the first time, we are essentially meeting a stranger. Did some of us grow them in our bodies? Yes. But that doesn't mean we know them. We are handed adorable little people formed precisely over nine months, but we don't know their preferences, we don't know how to soothe them or feed them or what will make them laugh. And this unknowing is exactly what shakes the confidence of many moms.

Luckily, we can distinguish between maternal instinct and the learned maternal behaviors of early parenthood. Let's think about early motherhood as a dynamic set of learned skills that continues to evolve through experience and adaptation as we get to know our babies rather than just relying on innate knowledge. If we frame motherhood as about learning, unlearning, and relearning, an experience shaped by trial, error, and our own willingness to adapt to both our child's needs and our own evolving identity, these skills might come to mind:

- Learning to understand our baby's cues.
- Learning to understand our baby's needs and how to meet them.
- Learning to soothe and comfort our babies.
- Learning to create a safe environment for ourselves and our babies.
- Learning how to balance our needs with the needs of those around us.

Let's compare that to what we might think of when we define "maternal instinct":

- An immediate, overwhelming love and desire to protect.
- An intuitive and immediate understanding of our child's needs.
- The innate ability to nurture and care for our children.
- Immediate ability and desire for selflessness and sacrifice.

If you look at these two lists, you can see that they are mostly identical, but one focuses on learned skills and the other focuses on assumed ability. Using the latter to frame caregiving creates immense pressure and self-doubt for mothers who don't experience an instant or magical connection to their babies.

What if, instead of telling new moms that their instincts will kick in and they'll know what to do, we told new moms that there is a learning curve? And that maternal behaviors are made up of bonding, learning, practice, and a few biological cues?

Charlie's Story

Charlie had always dreamt of being a mom, and she couldn't wait for her baby to arrive. When her son, Adam, was born, Charlie was thrilled. She had read the books, taken the birthing class, and felt as prepared as she could be for postpartum. After Adam was born, Charlie struggled. She found herself having difficulty soothing her baby. She was overwhelmed, exhausted, and she felt inadequate.

She had assumed that soothing her baby would be an innate maternal ability, and she told herself things like *This should be easy. This should come naturally to me. I'm failing because I'm struggling.* She had always believed that mothers were naturally equipped to care for their babies. Charlie felt like she was failing at the most basic tasks of motherhood. She questioned all her decisions, second-guessed her instincts, and felt massive waves of guilt. And she had intrusive thoughts on a loop: *What if I drop the baby, what if we get in a car accident, what if I fall down the stairs?* And *Did I lock the door, did I turn off the stove, is my hair straightener still plugged in, can the baby reach anything dangerous?*

She shared that she had attempted to ask her support system to normalize her hardships, and she was met with responses like "You'll figure it out," "You'll get the hang of it," or "Just trust your instincts." But when Charlie checked in with her instincts, she came up with nothing but worry. This made her feel embarrassed, caused her to doubt herself, and continued to fuel feelings of failure and isolation.

Charlie told me that she thought she had made a mistake and that maybe she wasn't cut out for motherhood. I introduced her to the idea of maternal behaviors as a set of learned skills, and Charlie began to identify all the ways that she was already practicing maternal behaviors.

Within a few weeks, Charlie began to understand that the learned skills of early parenthood were the skills she had always attributed to natural maternal instinct. And then she began to accept her challenges as learning curves instead of failures. With time, she was able to name the things she was doing daily that made her feel incredibly proud, and she was able to acknowledge that she was providing wonderful care for her baby. She began to combine her abilities with her drive for strengthening her skills in caregiving, and she was able to not only move forward from the idea that she had to be perfect but also, more important, embrace the idea that there is only one right way to be a mom.

Charlie came to realize that the myth of perfection and the myth of instant maternal instinct had damaged her confidence, and we worked on building that confidence back up. These myths that she believed had created unrealistic expectations and strong feelings of inadequacy that initially prevented her from seeking support and kept her from parenting in her own way. And that's okay. We normalized the struggle, and we also emphasized that her efforts were her successes.

If you, like Charlie, find yourself in a loop of not feeling nurturing enough, maternal enough, or good enough to parent your child, I'll offer you this: Research has shown that maternal behavior (yes, behavior) is shaped by an interplay of biological, psychological, and social factors. Innate maternal instinct as a set of untapped abilities is not supported by scientific evidence. I always understand a mom's desire to do their best while simultaneously encouraging them to talk to themselves nicely and grant themselves grace. If you find you're being too hard on yourself, you're allowed to take a break from the pressure.

Let's look closer at where this myth comes from. The idea of maternal instinct has evolved significantly over time, shaped by cultural, scientific, and societal influences.

Understanding the Stories We've Absorbed

Throughout history, motherhood has been viewed as a woman's inherent role, largely tied to her biological ability to bear children. This belief has been reinforced across civilizations by everything from ancient philosophy to religious doctrine and political structures.

The philosopher Aristotle asserted that "the male is by nature superior, and the female inferior . . . the one rules, and the other is ruled" (*Politics*, Book I). He argued that women's primary function was reproduction and child-rearing, positioning them as passive participants in society while men engaged in all of the governing, rule-making, and intellectual pursuits. Similar ideas were echoed in Roman society, where a woman's primary virtue was *pietas*—devotion to family and domestic duties.

Religious traditions have also shaped these expectations. In medieval Christian theology, thinkers like Thomas Aquinas built on Aristotle's views, teaching that women were divinely designed for nurturing roles. Biblical passages such as Titus 2:4–5 urged women to be "keepers at home," reinforcing the notion that motherhood was their natural calling. Confucianism in China similarly emphasized the moral duty of women to serve as caretakers of the family, a role formalized in the *Three Obediences* doctrine, which dictated a woman's subservience first to her father, then her husband, and finally her son.

While assumed gender roles may seem straightforward, they obscure a critical question: If one half of society was responsible for bringing life into the world, why was the burden of raising and nurturing children placed almost exclusively on them? Though the term *maternal instinct* had not yet been coined, the expectation that women inherently knew how to mother was deeply ingrained. As a result, motherhood was not just a role but an obligation, inextricably linked to a woman's identity and the survival of her community.

It wasn't until the Enlightenment and the Victorian era that maternal instinct began to be formally described. Jean-Jacques Rousseau wrote about women's natural inclination toward nurturing in the eighteenth century, particularly in his work *Émile, or On Education* (published in 1762), where he argued that women were naturally suited for motherhood and childcare, reinforcing the idea that their primary role was to raise and educate children. His views significantly influenced Enlightenment thinking about gender roles and the "natural" differences between men and women. This is also a key moment that society reinforced and upheld the idea of a "natural mother," devoted, moral, and self-sacrificing.

Fast-forward to the early twentieth century, when maternal behaviors became a subject less of assumption and more of medical and scientific study. Psychologists and ethologists like John Bowlby, who focused on attachment theory, emphasized the mother-child bond as vital to a child's development. These new areas of study reinforced the idea of a biological maternal instinct.

Then came the Industrial Revolution, 1760–1840, and the first wave of feminism, 1840–1920, which introduced voices that would challenge the idea of a natural mother as a fixed biological truth. Feminist thinkers like Simone de Beauvoir argued that maternal instinct was as much a social construct as it was biological, questioning the belief that women were born naturally predisposed to motherhood. This led to a growing recognition that maternal behaviors could be learned, influenced by social expectations and shaped by individual choice.

After looking at the history of bonding and the views of the mother's role, we can see that society has put a strong emphasis on the bond between a biological mother and her child as the "primary" relationship, suggesting that other bonds are secondary or somehow less important or significant. This idea is outdated AF and doesn't account for the fact that not all kids are brought home to a nuclear family. Children can and do form strong and healthy bonds with an array of caregivers, and it is unrealistic to assume that the only person naturally capable of caring for a new baby is their biological mother.

While a mother-child bond matters, biology isn't the only way a child forms a meaningful connection to their caregivers. Families come in countless configurations, and the bonds that hold them together aren't limited to the birthing parent and the baby. Data suggest that only about 46 percent of US households consist of two married parents with children—meaning that the majority, 54 percent of households, do not follow the nuclear family structure. Other family types include single-parent households, multigenerational families, cohabitating couples with children, families with same-sex parents, and other arrangements like grandparents raising grandchildren.

Caregiving, at its core, is about moments of connection, hours spent soothing, playing, and feeding, the daily rhythms of a life and love shared between a baby and their caregiver. Today we recognize caregiving as far more nuanced than either pure biology or pure social expectation. While biology certainly influences maternal behavior—hormonal changes during pregnancy and postpartum being notable examples—the idea that all women have an instant instinct to mother continues to be studied. And studies are revealing that caring for a baby is more than a set of instincts but is instead a collection of skills acquired through personal experiences, education, and support. As we peel back the layers of what makes a natural mother, we'll see it's more an interplay of nature, nurture, and personal experience than any of those one factors alone.

How Past Trauma Impacts the Ability to Bond

Understanding the impacts of previous traumas will help you recognize that struggling with maternal behaviors is common when you've experienced trauma in your past. There are several ways that trauma may come into play if you are struggling to bond with your baby:

- **Having a baby may activate your survival mode.** Trauma, especially unresolved trauma, can keep new parents in a state of constant hypervigilance or survival mode. This can make it hard for the nervous system to fully relax and engage in nurturing. A heightened state of stress or anxiety makes it harder for you to tune in to the cues of your newborn if you're trying hard to manage your own overwhelming emotions or psychological responses.

- **Having a baby may trigger your avoidance of big feelings.** Caretaking requires openness and vulnerability, but trauma survivors often develop coping mechanisms that can make intimacy feel unsafe or overwhelming. The intense attachment and dependency a baby demands can almost feel threatening for someone who has experienced relational trauma, like neglect or abuse, making bonding challenging.
- **Having a baby may bring on postpartum mood disorder.** We'll get into the full scope of perinatal mood disorders in Chapter 9, but trauma survivors are at a higher risk for postpartum mood disorders. When perinatal mood disorders are present, it can cause moms to feel detached or distant, posing a challenge in bonding.
- **Having a baby can trigger traumatic body memories.** Physical aspects of birth and then caring for a newborn, like breastfeeding, can trigger body memories of trauma. For some women, the physical sensations of feeding, holding, and being close to another body can bring up incredibly uncomfortable memories or feelings. This is particularly relevant for survivors of sexual trauma and can complicate the bonding experience.

If reading this made you feel like you've just been hit by a bus, please, please remember that a history of trauma does not mean that you can't or won't bond with your baby. It means that parts of postpartum might feel incredibly triggering or difficult. You are 100 percent capable of caring for your baby, and your baby is completely capable of bonding to you.

Check out Appendix B (page 261) for some great resources to help unpack a history or trauma or abuse.

Hormones and Bonding

After birth, a mother's body and brain undergo an incredible hormonal transformation that primes her for bonding. In the days surrounding childbirth, our baby-growing hormones drop dramatically. The sharp decline is one of the steepest hormonal changes a human can experience, especially considering it affects multiple body systems, emotions, and behaviors.

While the hormonal shifts that happen after childbirth are significant, they don't turn us into experts on caregiving who automatically know how to change a diaper or interpret every cry. It's still only part of the full picture. But each hormone and brain area plays a unique role that aids us in caregiving and bonding, priming our system to learn and finely tune our abilities for maternal responsiveness, attachment, and resilience.

Key hormones like oxytocin (the "love hormone") enhance bonding and promote caregiving behaviors, while prolactin boosts our sensitivity to our baby's needs, making us more attuned to their cues. Estrogen and progesterone help shape the brain for responsiveness, and dopamine reinforces positive caregiving behaviors by rewarding us when a baby smiles. Serotonin, which helps stabilize our mood, is crucial for navigating the emotional roller coaster of postpartum life. Meanwhile, areas in our brain like the medial preoptic area and the amygdala guide us in responding to our baby's needs and processing emotions.

But none of these hormones or parts of our brain inherently teaches us the practical skills of parenting. While they certainly set the stage for care, true maternal expertise comes through experience and learning, not instinct alone.

And although biological factors such as hormonal changes and neurological responses weave into the mix that shapes caregiving behaviors, they 1,000 percent do not tell the full story of parental bonding and attachment. Parental love and responsiveness are *not* exclusive to biological mothers or fathers.

Sophia's Story

Sophia came to meet me shortly after the birth of her and her wife's first baby. Sophia's wife, Jenna, had had a smooth pregnancy and was feeling good postpartum—she felt she was learning the skills she needed and felt comfortable listening to her instincts. Sophia, on the other hand, did not feel connected to her parental instincts even slightly. She was watching her wife, who, after carrying and birthing their baby, seemed to be having a seamless time bonding, and Sophia felt like she was losing not only her wife but also any possibility of bonding as a primary caregiver.

Sophia and I started to explore what being a "natural mother" meant to her and what was happening to make her feel on the outside of her family unit. This is a super-common experience for a noncarrying partner.

In this particular case, one of our goals was to help Sophia unlearn her ideas of what a mother should be, learn what she wanted motherhood to look like for her, and then create the steps she could take to work on developing her own unique caregiving blueprint for her and her baby.

We started small. I encouraged Sophia to begin creating daily routines to focus on one-on-one bonding for her and her baby. In this particular family, they started with bath time and bedtime every night. Sophia tackled bath time and bedtime solo with a bottle, and it went great. Sophia began to feel the bond with her baby, and Jenna was able to start going to bed earlier and felt slightly more rested when she started her day.

Sophia came to embrace the tiny moments of connection and became undoubtedly bonded with her baby. The acts of care that she began practicing every day turned into sacred time with her baby and a feeling of inclusion in her family. Within a few months, Sophia began to feel more relaxed and sentimental in the way she talked about both her wife and their child. The emotional hollowness that she had been feeling had been replaced by a deep and growing love that didn't rely on biology but was instead built on loving moments.

Sophia learned that love doesn't have a specific starting line or finish line. Love unfolded in its own time, and she discovered her natural motherhood. She learned the areas of caregiving that she appreciated, she found the ways that she and her partner could complement each other in their unique ways of mothering, and she came to understand herself as capable of meeting the needs of her baby.

The Truth About Caregiving

Understanding that bonding with one's baby isn't solely confined to biological mothers or even traditional family structures gives us a more inclusive framework for what it means to parent a child. Families, no matter the form, are capable of providing the love and security that a baby needs, and the myth of the "ideal" family fades when we acknowledge that a bond between people can grow in many ways.

To build a new cultural understanding around the learned skills of caretaking, it feels important that we start by letting go of rigid and idealized standards that assume caregiving and the learned art of mothering happen instantaneously or in a specific way. When we look at motherhood as only a blend of born biological ability, societal expectations, and cultural myths, we fail to represent the diversity of family structures and parental experiences that many of us exist in. When we reinforce that so much of motherhood happens gradually and is a flexible process, we can begin to foster a cultural shift that recognizes caretaking as a community job and not just a mom's job.

Ultimately, changing the cultural narrative around what caring for a baby means allows us to redefine what it is to be a "good parent." To support new parents, we need to affirm that many of the skills of parenting are not born when our baby is born. Taking a more flexible approach and understanding allows us to be more at ease and prouder of our own experiences. As we continue to cultivate a more fluid understanding, we can shift our expectations to focus on taking our own pace with curiosity rather than self-criticism or judgment.

Let's shift away from the idea that a mom is the only one who has the natural skills to parent based on instinct and begin to explore the idea of bonding as a shared and family responsibility. Instead of looking at bonding as the job of mom, let's look at ways that we can focus on creating authentic parental bonds for everyone in the family. The truth is that instinct can be a shared experience. Instead of looking at nurturing as solely an inherent female trait, we will explore how everyone who cares for babies can develop nurturing instincts.

Road Map to Change: Learning the Art of Noticing

When you're a new mom, the myth of the natural mother can feel huge, unattainable, and very vague. You're handed this tiny, fragile human and expected to just know what to do—except many new parents don't know what to do. And that's not a personal failure. It's a societal failure rooted in unrealistic expectations about motherhood.

Our truth is that caring for a baby isn't something you're born knowing; it's something you learn. Just like any other skill, it takes time, practice, and a lot of trial and error. Yet we continue to embrace a culture that sells the idea that maternal instinct is a magical, innate force that should guide us through postpartum.

This road map is about breaking up with this myth. It's about normalizing the learning curve of motherhood, giving yourself permission to ask for help, and creating systems of support that allow you to thrive.

This chapter's Road Map to Change is twofold. If we want to begin understanding motherhood as a combination of learned skills, hormonal shifts, and cultural expectations, we have to talk about the learning process as well as create support for new parents. We're going to start by reflecting on our wins and continue by beginning a practice in the art of noticing.

Road Map to Change Exercises

REFLECTING ON YOUR WINS

As you go through this road map, start by flipping the script on what it means to "get it right." Instead of aiming for perfection, focus on growth by taking time to reflect on your wins during postpartum.

This is a perfect time to get your journal. Use the reflection questions I've provided for each win, or write down your own notes.

You're going to practice noticing. Noticing is about being fully present and attuned to the small, subtle moments between you and your baby. When we focus on noticing, we shift our mindset from expectations and pressure to simply being open to observing the moment we're in. We have to be able to notice the small bonding moments before we can celebrate them.

The First Purposeful Eye Contact

The first time you noticed your baby gazing lovingly back at you is a huge bonding moment! Eye contact is a key way babies begin to recognize and trust caregivers. This is one of your baby's earliest ways of communicating.

Reflection Questions

1. What does it feel like to know your baby is seeing you?
2. How do you think these moments of connection help you better understand and care for your baby?
3. In what ways does this milestone reflect your baby's growing trust in you as a caregiver?

Soothing Moments That Are Coming More Naturally

You know those moments when you're able to calm a baby without much stress? Yep, you're building the foundation of a great mom in calming your baby during fussy moments. This security is the foundation for attachment.

Reflection Questions

1. How has your confidence grown as you've learned to calm your baby during fussy moments?
2. What approaches have you discovered that work well to calm your baby that you also love?
3. How do these soothing moments deepen your bond and build trust between you and your baby?

When Your Baby Smiles at You

Seeing your baby respond to you with a smile is probably one of the greatest moments in parenthood. The reciprocal smile is a small but mighty way our babies begin to show social engagement, making you finally feel connected and appreciated. This is when so many moms begin to feel like all the hard work of postpartum is worth it.

Reflection Questions

1. What emotions do you experience when your baby starts to smile at you?
2. How does your baby's smile encourage and motivate you during the challenging moments of postpartum?
3. What does your baby's smile teach you about the power of connection and communication, even without words?

Establishing a Routine Together

Creating small but steady routines around feeding, diaper changes, and bedtime rituals helps you and your baby become familiar with what your life together looks like. Repeating daily routines builds trust, security, and togetherness. In our house, my husband took bath time and story time. Our kids still love this routine, and my husband still loves this bonding time with our kids.

Reflection Questions

1. How have daily routines helped you and your baby feel more connected and secure?
2. What part of your routine feels the most special or enjoyable for you and your baby?

3. How do you see these early routines shaping your family's sense of togetherness?

Skin-to-Skin

A baby who doesn't want to sleep alone can feel incredibly overwhelming, and skin-to-skin moments are invaluable in maintaining that safe space that makes a mom feel like a mom. Babywearing is my favorite skin-to-skin hack; that way I don't feel nap trapped and am still able to give the baby the closeness they need with my free hands to get stuff done—or not, but at the very least I'm not stuck under a sleeping babe. Cuddling, babywearing, and soothing with touch release oxytocin, deepening our developing bond as the person of comfort and connection for our baby.

Reflection Questions

1. How do skin-to-skin moments with your baby make you feel as a mom?
2. What benefits have you noticed for both you and your baby during skin-to-skin time?
3. How has incorporating babywearing or similar practices helped you balance meeting your baby's needs with your own?

When You and Your Baby Begin to Respond to Each Other

When your baby is wailing and you've learned to decipher between hungry cries and tired cries, this is bonding! When your baby is in their little bouncy chair and laughing while you're showering or engaged in your conversation while you're on the phone, this is them noticing you the way you've been seeing them. You noticing them, them noticing you, the mutual trust you're beginning to build—that is bonding.

Reflection Questions

1. How has learning to interpret your baby's cues (like hunger or tiredness) changed the way you feel about your bond with them?
2. What moments of mutual engagement—like your baby laughing with you or noticing you—have stood out the most?
3. How does the growing trust between you and your baby shape the way you interact with each other?

Experiencing Comfort as a Caregiver

I get asked all of the time by postpartum moms if motherhood will get easier, to which I usually respond, "The challenges change, but you'll get more confident and comfortable in the role." Feeling more at ease and confident in caregiving will continue to build mutual trust, support relaxation in motherhood, and help you create the calm you want.

Reflection Questions

1. In what areas of motherhood do I feel most at ease, and what routines or practices have helped me feel more confident in those moments?
2. How can you start to embrace the challenges of motherhood as opportunities for growth rather than signs of inadequacy?
3. What small steps can you take to create a more relaxed and trusting environment for both yourself and your baby, even when things feel overwhelming?

Are you feeling a little bit better now about maternal instinct and the myths around bonding? I hope so. Because that's the goal.

Three Important Things

1. Bonding takes time.
2. You aren't doing anything wrong. Promise.
3. You are exactly the mom your baby needs. You're learning, and sometimes growth comes with growing pains.

What's next? My question for you: When I say *attachment*, what is the first word that comes to your mind?

5

The Myth of the Perfect Mom-Baby Attachment

When I ask parents their hopes for their child, the answers are generally the same:

1. Parents want their kids to be happy.
2. Parents want their kids to be healthy.
3. Parents want their kids to grow up and have healthy and supportive relationships.

As new parents, we want to feel like we're doing our best in all areas of caring for our babies to make sure that they have the best possible adulthood with the tools we've given them. And we know that this starts with their relationship with us. The mother-child relationship becomes the cornerstone, or the foundation, for our children's emotional intelligence—and that's a *lot* of pressure.

Most of us have heard the term *attachment parenting*, but we don't know what it means. We know that a secure attachment is the goal, but we also don't know what that means or how to get it.

Here's the thing about attachment: It's a psychological theory that has gone mainstream, but for many of us, its meaning and application remain hard to understand. If you've ever heard the term *attachment parenting* and immediately panicked, wondering if you're messing up your child with an unhealthy attachment, take a deep breath. You aren't alone. That creeping sense of inadequacy? It's fed by our fifth myth: the myth of the perfect attachment.

Attachment theory, when boiled down to its essence, is about connection. It's the science of how relationships form, develop, and are sustained over time. But what does it look like in real life? How does it show up in the blurs of early parenting, when the baby's crying and you're just trying to finish one cup of coffee? To understand this, we first need to demystify what attachment means and what it doesn't.

Even with a background in counseling psychology, it took me years to feel confident teaching new moms about attachment theory. It's one thing to categorize attachment styles in the textbooks—secure, avoidant, anxious, disorganized—but it's another to live the experience of forming healthy attachments. This is mostly because attachment isn't a static concept. It's not something you achieve and check off a list. Instead, it's an ongoing and evolving process. It's shaped by daily interaction, being present in the ups and downs of living life with a baby, and, most importantly, your willingness to reflect and adapt.

For many of us, understanding attachment begins with looking inward and then backward at our own history. How did our own caregivers model connection? Did we feel safe, seen, and supported as children? Or did we grow up feeling uncertain, overlooked, or dismissed? These early experiences shape our attachment styles, which in turn influence how we approach relationships as adults—including the relationships we form with our children.

The myth of the perfect attachment adds an extra layer of pressure to the already complex dynamic of becoming a mom. It whispers *If you don't get this right, you're failing your child.* But attachment isn't about getting it right all of the time. It's about being good enough most of the time. For any perfectionist, that might sound like a low bar, but "good enough" parenting is a concept rooted in decades of research. It means showing up, being present, and meeting your baby's needs to the best of your ability—most of the time. Not all of the time, because that isn't realistic.

And attachment theory isn't just about moms. Attachment isn't a one-way street. It's a relationship. It's about the interplay between you and your baby, the dance of connection and response. When your baby cries and you comfort them, you're building attachment. When they coo and you smile back, you're building attachment. When you're too tired to do anything but hold them and whisper, "I'm here and I love you," you're building attachment. These moments, small as they may seem, are the foundation of a secure relationship.

Building a healthy attachment also means taking care of your own well-being so you can show up for your baby in meaningful ways. You can't pour from an empty cup, and you can't pour from a broken cup. This might mean revisiting your own childhood experiences to better understand how they're influencing your parenting today. It's not selfish to do your own work; it's necessary.

One of the most freeing truths about attachment is that it's a long game. It's not defined by a single moment or a single mistake. It's the cumulative effect of countless interactions over time. This means that if you have a rough day (or week, or month), it's okay. Repair is a crucial part of attachment. When you acknowledge missteps, apologize if needed, and recommit to showing up, you're teaching your child one of the most valuable lessons they can learn: Relationships can survive imperfection.

So what does this mean for you as a new mom? It means letting go of the myth of the perfect attachment. It means embracing the messy, imperfect reality of building a relationship with your child. And it means trusting yourself and trusting that the love you're providing is enough—even on the days you feel like you're failing.

As you read this chapter, my goal is that you'll find clarity, reassurance, and maybe even a little bit of energy in the joy of attachment. Let's break down the myths, explore science, and discover what it really means to build a secure, loving connection with your child. Because attachment isn't about perfection. It's about showing up, learning, and growing together.

What Is Attachment Theory?

John Bowlby was a British psychiatrist who developed attachment theory, which emphasizes that infants form close relationships with primary caregivers, usually their mothers, to ensure survival and promote healthy emotional and social development. Bowlby believed that these early bonds are crucial for emotional security.

Attachment theory explains how early relationships shape a child's sense of security and ability to trust others. The way a caregiver responds to their baby's needs plays a significant role in shaping attachment, but it's important to remember that attachment is not about perfection—it's about patterns of care over time.

The main takeaways of Bowlby's attachment theory are:

1. Children between six months and thirty months are likely to form emotional attachments to familiar caregivers—particularly those who are responsive to the child's cues.
2. Events that interfere with attachment—abrupt separation, inability of caregivers to be responsive—have both short-term and longer-term negative impacts on the child's emotional healing and cognitive development.
3. The formation of emotional attachments creates the foundation for personality and emotional development.

4. The emotional attachments of young children are shown in their preferences for particular people and their ability to use these adults as a secure base.

Let's take a look at the different types of attachment that make up Bowlby's attachment theory.

The Four Types of Attachment

Here are the four main attachment styles and what they mean for parenting:

1. **Secure attachment:** Babies develop secure attachment when their caregivers respond to their needs with warmth, consistency, and reliability. A securely attached baby trusts that their caregiver will comfort and support them, leading to confidence and emotional resilience as they grow.
2. **Anxious attachment:** This can develop when a caregiver is inconsistent—sometimes responsive, sometimes unavailable. Babies with anxious attachment may become clingy, distressed when separated, or overly focused on seeking reassurance. Parents don't cause this by occasionally missing a cue, but if unpredictability is a constant, babies can struggle with trust.
3. **Avoidant attachment:** Babies with avoidant attachment learn that expressing their needs doesn't always lead to comfort, so they appear independent and may not seek help when distressed. This can develop when caregivers discourage emotional expression or frequently prioritize independence over connection.
4. **Disorganized attachment:** This often results from inconsistent, chaotic, or frightening caregiving. Babies with disorganized attachment show mixed behaviors—

seeking comfort but also appearing fearful of their caregiver—because their source of security has also been a source of stress.

Building a Healthy Attachment With Your Baby

In reading through the different types of attachment, maybe you are now working to figure out what your own attachment style is. You might also be wondering *How do I heal my own learned attachment style to ensure my baby forms a secure attachment to me?* If you're asking that, you aren't alone. If you've ever thought *I'm not going to do _____ like my parents did* or *I'm terribly afraid that I'm going to mess up my kid because I never had secure attachment when I was little*, that's completely understandable. Our attachment styles can drive our behavior, and none of us want to make the same mistakes we think our parents made.

The truth is, attachment styles are not fixed but instead are dynamic patterns that can change and adapt over time. Recognizing the influence of our own early caregivers is important, but it's equally important to understand that both we and our children have the capacity to evolve. One small mistake isn't going to destroy your child's ability to form secure attachments. Even if you were a child who developed attachment patterns that felt less than ideal, there's always the opportunity to nurture change and build healthier and more secure connections.

Secure attachment is built through everyday moments of care, connection, and repair. Babies don't need perfect parents; they need *good enough* parents who consistently try to meet their needs and respond with love. Here are some ways you can develop secure attachment with your baby.

- **Attunement matters more than perfection.** Your baby doesn't need you to catch every cue instantly. What matters is that you *try* to respond, and when you miss something, you make up for it with comfort and care.

- **Repair is powerful.** If you have a tough day (or week), the opportunity to repair—by soothing, reconnecting, and being present—matters more than the original misstep.
- **Trust is built over time.** One rough night, a missed feeding cue, or a moment of frustration won't determine your baby's attachment style. What counts is the overall pattern of care.

The myth that "one wrong move" will harm your child's attachment is one of the most harmful messages new parents absorb. In reality, attachment is a process, not a pass-fail test. Showing up, responding with warmth, and offering comfort—even imperfectly—is what truly builds a secure bond.

Attachment Style Takeaways

Graduate school taught that sometimes too much information is too much information. That said, I want to provide you each with a few bite-sized takeaways and actionable insights for each attachment style.

- **Secure attachment:** Secure attachment is built on a foundation of trust and responsiveness. The early postpartum period is the perfect time to begin building this foundation. Small, consistent acts like responding to our babies' cries help to convey that we are safe, loving, and will show up.
- **Anxious attachment:** Anxious attachment can develop when caregiving is inconsistent, leaving the baby unsure about whether their needs will be

met. By focusing on our actions rather than getting lost in our emotions during postpartum, we can work toward establish predictability in our responses to our babies.

- **Avoidant attachment:** Avoidant attachment forms when a baby learns that their caregiver may not respond to their needs, leading them to suppress their emotional expressions. In the earliest days of motherhood, we're still learning how to care for our babies, and it's normal to miss cues while we're learning to interpret our newborns signals. The key is to prioritize responding, even if we feel uncertain about what our baby needs. Holding, cuddling, and talking to our baby—especially during the calm moments—can help foster a sense of secure connection.
- **Disorganized attachment:** Disorganized attachment arises when caregivers are both a source of comfort and fear, often due to their own experiences as a child. Recognizing early signs of stress or overwhelm in ourselves is crucial. Postpartum is naturally a vulnerable time, and leaning on our support systems can help create a more stable environment for both us and our babies. It's not about avoiding difficult emotions but ensuring that our big feelings don't translate into inconsistent care for our little ones.

Baby's Attachment Needs

When you first meet your newborn, you are quite literally at the very, very beginning of building the foundation of healthy attachment. The realities of bonding and attachment are far more nuanced than the romanticized version of postpartum that many new moms are used to seeing. A perfect storm of evolutionary theories, cultural portrayals, and traditional gender roles have created a space where many new moms feel like they're failing if they don't feel an instant attachment. So what does attachment look like, anyway? What do our newborns need from us in terms of safety, security, and consistency?

Picture your newborn, a teeny tiny little person full of needs and potential. In these early months, the fourth trimester specifically, caregivers play a crucial role in laying the foundation for what will become attachment. During this time, consistent responsiveness is the first step in building a strong attachment between mom and baby.

Around three months, babies start to recognize familiar faces, they begin to smile, and their smiles become more meaningful—and less about them passing gas. They may begin to show preferences for certain people, or they may not; they are still very little.

As a baby reaches six months, their attachment becomes more focused. Around this time infants begin to turn to specific caregivers for comfort, protection, and reassurance. This is when they want mama, and mama knows it. By nine months, babies are becoming more independent, exploring their surroundings. While they become little explorers, they remain attached to their primary caregivers—this is the period of time that they form bonds with those who respond warmly and consistently to their needs.

Between eighteen months and three years, caregivers become the home base. Through their interactions, children have developed a sense of safety and security, which is crucial to their emotional development, self-esteem, and positive relationships.

Bari's Story

Bari came to see me for the first time when she was six months pregnant. "My parents were awful, and I'm afraid I'm going to be awful too," she shared during our intake session. Over the next few weeks, Bari and I explored the parts of her childhood she was afraid of repeating when she became a mom. She shared that she grew up in a very religious home with traditional values and that as the daughter of the family, she was held to very different standards than those placed on her brothers. Bari described her relationship with her parents in a way that matched disorganized attachment.

She told me that her mother could be warm and loving one moment and cold and punishing the next. Her father, though less volatile, was distant—present in the home but emotionally absent. "I never knew what version of my mom I was going to get," Bari admitted. "One day she would praise me for setting the table perfectly. The next, she would scream at me for something small, like forgetting to refill the salt shaker. It made me feel like I was always walking on eggshells."

As Bari's pregnancy progressed, so did our work together. Bari was deeply afraid of becoming her mother, of unintentionally making her own child feel the same instability she had endured. "I don't want my baby to be afraid of me," she said, her voice shaking. "But what if I don't know how to be different?"

We talked a lot about the power of awareness—how recognizing patterns is the first step to breaking them. We explored what safety in a parent-child relationship actually looks like, and I reminded her that secure attachment isn't about being a perfect mother; it's about being a consistent, responsive one.

One session, Bari came in with a journal she had been keeping throughout our work together. She flipped to a page where she had written *I can be warm and consistent. I can be different.* She smiled, a little unsure but hopeful. "I've been practicing responding to myself with kindness when I get overwhelmed," she told me. "I figure if I can do that for me, I can do it for my baby too."

After her baby was born, Bari and I continued our sessions. She had moments of doubt, like all new parents do, but she also had something she had never experienced as a child—self-compassion. One day she shared an experience that made us both pause.

"The other night, my baby wouldn't stop crying. I tried everything—feeding, rocking, swaddling. Nothing worked. I started feeling that old panic rise in my chest, the same feeling I had as a kid when my mom would get angry. But then I remembered what you and I talked about, how I don't have to be perfect—I just have to show up."

She took a deep breath and continued. "So I held her, even though I didn't have the answer. I whispered, 'I know, baby. I know it's hard. I'm here.' And eventually, she settled. And so did I."

Bari looked at me, tears in her eyes. "That moment—it was everything. Because for the first time in my life, I wasn't afraid of being a mother. I *was* a mother."

And in that moment, she wasn't just breaking cycles—she was building something new.

Recognizing Attachment Styles

When moms show up in my office concerned that their attachment style is harming their baby, I usually end up at the same place: How are parents supposed to recognize their own attachment style if they haven't been taught anything about them? And why isn't attachment talked about as an ongoing process rather than something that happens immediately, at first glance?

A quick scroll through social media can leave even the most highly educated parenting expert wondering if their own attachment style is normal. The myth of the perfect attachment will leave any unknowing postpartum parent feeling awful when they're handed their new baby, and it will feel overwhelming instead of magical. The moment where a postpartum mom thinks holding her baby is supposed to be "attached at first sight" and is surprised when it's not, is the exact spot where the real postpartum experience meets the myth of the perfect attachment. Many new moms believe that if they have an immediate attachment to their baby, then they're a good mom, and if they don't feel instantly connected, then there's something wrong.

Over the years, I've been welcomed into the homes of many new parents, and I've been asked many times if I felt attached to my babies when I first laid eyes on them. I've sat with moms who are days into motherhood, sleep deprived and already concerned that they're messing up their little baby because they don't feel attached to them.

While I've typically been asked, "When did you feel attached/bonded to your baby?" and "Did you experience love at first sight?" what I've come to learn is that these questions are a way to hide behind the one question that moms actually want to ask *Is there something wrong with me because I love my baby but don't really feel that unbreakable bond that everyone talks about?* What most moms are seeking to understand is if they are bonding with their baby "the right way."

Love and Attachment Aren't the Same Thing

Loving your new baby and having a healthy attachment with your baby are related but not the same thing. They both involve emotional dynamics and connection but present differently.

When we think of love, we think of the emotional affection and care a parent feels for their child. This love can be immediate, it can grow with time, and it usually encompasses some desire to nurture, protect, and provide for our baby's well-being.

When we think of attachment, we either have absolutely no idea what it means or we think of a more complex process that develops over time through consistent, responsive caregiving. It's harder to explain what attachment *feels* like, but it can be described loosely as a bond based on trust, security, and a sense of safety.

Love arises spontaneously, while attachment is built through a series of interactions over time. Love is a feeling of affection, while attachment is the specific bond you have with your baby. Love feels more immediate and more emotional, whereas attachment is gradual and more in our heads—it's a more cognitive process.

While love and attachment in parenthood are intertwined, they are different and distinct concepts. Moving forward, we can think of love as the emotional foundation of motherhood while attachment is the (hopefully healthy) bond that will grow with time, consistency, and care. Understanding this difference, for me, helped me appreciate the different ways that we can connect with our babies to cultivate strong and secure relationships.

Because let's be honest—we know that we love our babies, and separating love from bonding is bound to boost the confidence of a new mom.

When we're in the depths of postpartum and caught up in the emotional intensity of caring for a new baby, sometimes it's hard to remember that bonding takes time, and therefore attachment will take time as well. It can feel incredibly hard to feel connected to a little person who doesn't smile yet, isn't making eye contact, and doesn't let you sleep.

The myth of immediate and perfect attachment has brought countless moms to my office saying they don't want to mess up like their own parents did and asking for a clearer understanding of what healthy attachment is and how it can be achieved with a six-day-old baby.

New moms asking me about my own experiences in early motherhood demonstrates an absolute need for reassurance, a desire to know that their postpartum experience isn't abnormal. These mothers are seeking permission to feel what they feel instead of what they believe they should be feeling. My response to these questions is usually some variety of "the mother-child bond is really powerful, and attachment takes time."

The myth of a perfect attachment between mother and baby directly impacts how mothers perceive themselves and how they feel they are being perceived by others, creating a pressure to display a certain type of bond with their newborn. This pressure can begin right at birth, when hospitals, birthing centers, health care providers, and visitors weigh in on how a mother and baby should be bonding. Health care environments like Baby-Friendly Hospitals can play a significant role in shaping a new mom's self-confidence.

Baby-Friendly Hospitals are health care facilities that adhere to specific practices and policies designed to support breastfeeding and improve maternal and infant care. I gave birth to both of my babies in a Baby-Friendly Hospital.

In practice, what this looks like is in-room breastfeeding support, breastfeeding education, and "rooming-in," the term used for babies being in the room with their caregivers instead of the baby being taken to a nursery. And while the intentions behind such initiatives are positive—encouraging breastfeeding and supporting maternal care—they can inadvertently amplify the expectation of immediate attachment, reinforcing the idea that there is a right or wrong way to bond with a newborn. And these policies don't take into account the diversity of birthing experiences, surrogacy, adoption, and the many ways that people become a family.

Having a preemie in a baby-friendly hospital gave me additional insights into the judgment new moms face around bonding and attachment. In the NICU, I overheard nurses discussing mothers who hadn't visited or whose visits were sporadic. It was clear that bonding was being judged, as though time spent with the baby equated to love and a desire for new moms to mother.

In the NICU, I saw firsthand how quickly we judge a mother's love based on appearances—who visits the most, who looks the most confident, who seems to "get it" right away. But attachment doesn't work that way. It's not measured by how much skin-to-skin you do in those first twenty-four hours or whether you feel an immediate, overwhelming sense of connection. It's built through patience, presence, and practice.

With my son that first night in the hospital, I felt like a mom. The second night, I felt like a fraud. And the third night, I sobbed because I missed my dog. It took time to feel like *Jack's* mom. Time to understand his cries, trust myself, and settle into the role.

So if you're reading this and wondering whether you've *gotten it right* yet, I want you to know—you don't have to. Attachment isn't something you win or lose in a single moment. It's a relationship that grows as you do. And feeling like you have no idea what you're doing? That's just part of the process.

Nature's Bad Moms

I tell any new mom that comes to me with doubt, "The fact that you're trying is a sign of a wonderful mother." Being worried that you aren't doing well, as counterintuitive as it seems, is a sign that you're doing better than well. To make you feel a bit better, let's see how some of nature's worst moms parent.

1. Sea turtle moms lay their eggs in nests on the beach, and then they leave. Pop 'em out and head for the door. When the little baby sea turtles are born, they are left to fend for themselves.

2. Harp seal moms remain devoted and dedicated to their pups . . . for twelve full days. Harp babies are fed milk for the first twelve days of their lives, and around day twelve, that's it for mama-baby bonding. Mama seal takes off to go mate again, and the babies are left to figure the rest out.
3. Cuckoo mamas trick other birds into raising their kids. No joke. The cuckoo mom lays her eggs in the nest of another bird. And then she leaves.
4. Panda moms are pretty bad moms. Despite the fact that pandas often have twins, the mama panda will pick one of the twins to care for and abandon the other.
5. And lastly, the mama bear herself, the black bear, generally has two to three cubs at a time. And when she is given the gift of a singleton, the mama bear will often abandon it, deciding that raising only one baby isn't worth her time or energy.

So anytime you're questioning if your attachment is healthy, remember that you didn't pull any of the stunts that the moms above have.

The Truth About Attachment and Bonding

The myth of instant attachment paints a picture of motherhood that's beautiful, effortless, and, unfortunately, unrealistic. It places unnecessary pressure on mothers to feel an immediate and overwhelming relationship with their baby, leaving little room for the natural, messy, and deeply human process of getting to know each other. The truth is that attachment, like all meaningful relationships, takes time. It's not a moment but a series of moments—late-night feedings, quiet snuggles, and learning how to meet each other's needs.

By recognizing this, we free ourselves from the guilt and shame of not "feeling it" right away. We create space for the real work of building a connection: being present, responding to our baby's cues, and giving ourselves grace as we learn.

If you're feeling incredibly triggered or sad or heartbroken, I want to reassure you that healing the wounds of your own childhood and repairing the attachment injuries that you absorbed is totally possible. Any hurt that you've experienced doesn't mean that you're going to repeat any of what was done to you as a kid. Healing the mother's wound can be hard and heavy work. Although we will not be going deep into healing this aspect of attachment in this book, there are plenty of resources and supports you can connect with that can help you heal. At the end of this book, in Appendix B (page 261), you will find a list of my favorite resources.

For now, we're going to focus on what happens moving forward. Let's channel our energies into breaking cycles and building our own path toward healthy and secure attachments between ourselves and our babies.

Road Map to Change: Focusing on Actions

If someone had told you that at three months postpartum your baby isn't expected to show signs of attachment (affection, eye contact even), would you feel differently about your experience?

Let's start with ditching the idea that we should feel a certain way and instead lay a loving foundation by focusing on the tasks of caring for our baby: skin-to-skin time, feeding, responding to baby's cues, and practicing being present. It's the actions of early postpartum that build secure attachment.

The earliest days of postpartum are both beautiful and challenging. The journey of bonding with our baby can sometimes feel overshadowed by our own false pursuit of perfection. Attachment is a process that takes time and consistency, and during this time, if we shift our focus from feelings to actions, it can be transformative. While it's natural to feel overwhelmed with sleepless nights and physical recovery, the key in fostering secure attachment lies in the simple, intentional acts of caregiving.

Road Map to Change Exercises

Here are some exercises to help you focus on your actions first and emotions second. In each exercise, I encourage you to star, highlight, or mark up the scenario that feels most attainable for you.

INSTEAD OF OVERTHINKING, TRY RESPONDING

The scenario: Your baby is hysterically crying, and you are trying everything in your power to figure out what your baby needs. You're feeling frantic and overstimulated and just want the loud screams to stop so you can gather your frantic thoughts.

Try this:

1. Take five deep breaths, and if you need to, grab some sound-canceling headphones. Do what you need to do in the moment of chaos to ground yourself in any sort of calm.
2. Instead of being in your head trying to figure out what's wrong, put your energy into your actions. Try feeding, try bouncing, try going for a walk with the baby. Try a variety of actions until you can learn what this cry means.
3. The key here is showing up, remaining as calm as you can, and trying not to get carried away in your own worry.
4. This will take a lot of practice, but I promise you that you can meet the chaos of the moment with your calm.

INSTEAD OF CREATING A RIGID SCHEDULE, TRY CREATING MEANINGFUL ROUTINES

The scenario: You've started to make commitments outside of the house during the day with your baby, and then a sleep regression hits. Everyone had a hard night, and the thought of mom and baby music class sounds exhausting.

Try this: Grant yourself permission to be flexible. Rather than following a rigid schedule, especially in times that you know whatever is on the schedule is going to create stress for you, allow yourself the grace of being flexible so you can rest, baby can rest, and both you and baby can take time to recharge.

INSTEAD OF REACTING, TRY CLEAR COMMUNICATION

The scenario: You notice that your partner is also feeling overwhelmed. When they suggest a change in how you bathe the baby, you immediately feel defensive and want to start screaming insults back at them. You recognize that these are moments of high stress, but you also wish they would help instead of criticizing.

Try this: Instead of reacting immediately in anger (and I totally understand if that's your immediate reaction), try to work on practicing clear communication. Remember, just as attachment is going to take you time, it's also going to take time for your partner. You can start by using "I" statements and work as a team to foster a collaborative approach to caregiving.

INSTEAD OF AVOIDING ASKING FOR HELP, TRY EMBRACING SUPPORT

The scenario: Your partner has returned to work, and you're feeling overwhelmed with feelings of inadequacy but are having a hard time accepting help. You're still convinced that if you need help, you aren't good enough.

Try this: Instead of avoiding support, work toward embracing the support. If it's really challenging for you to ask for help, you could consider help days or help mornings where you have friends or family over. This not only alleviates your workload but also continues to build connections and reinforces that your baby has a whole community that loves them.

By shifting our focus from feelings to concrete actions, we not only give ourselves space and time to grow healthy attachments to our babies but also foster a more supportive and loving environment for ourselves. When mom is loved and cared for, she is all the more able to share her best self back.

Three Important Things

1. Understanding our own attachment style isn't about blaming but about understanding and healing. By addressing our own attachment styles, we are able to rewrite the narrative for future generations. Our attachment styles can be passed on, but they are not life sentences.
2. Attachment takes time. It's okay if you don't feel immediately bonded to your baby.
3. Focus on actions and not feelings in the early days of postpartum; your loving actions will lead to warm attachments.

What's coming next? I will leave you with this question: If you're being honest with yourself, how much have you enjoyed postpartum?

6

The Myth of "Mom" Being Your Only Identity

Becoming a mother might transform you—but it doesn't mean you just disappear. And yet so many new moms feel as though their entire identity has been erased the moment their baby arrives. This may be because the myth that once you become a mother, you are *only* a mother is woven into our culture, reinforced in subtle (and not-so-subtle) ways—how we talk about moms, what we expect of them, and how little space we leave for their dreams, desires, and individuality.

But here's the truth: Becoming a mother doesn't mean you cease to exist. It doesn't mean your passions, ambitions, and personality should take a back seat indefinitely.

And this is exactly where I tell you with my full heart and my greatest gusto: Postpartum isn't just about the baby, and it's okay if you're unsure how you feel about your identity as a new mom.

It's possible that twelve months ago you were planning a girls' trip, or taking a last-minute road trip or date night, or having a lazy morning. And now you're awake all night—and being awake all night sucks. Is it a special time when we can bond with our babies? Sure. But sleep deprivation sucks so hard that it can leave even moms who need little sleep (hi, it's me; I'm the problem) begging to any deity that will listen for more. Immense sleep deprivation can impact our physical health, mental health, clarity . . .

response time. And still, moms are told to soak up every moment of postpartum with joy and enthusiasm.

Cleaning bottles also sucks; so does getting pooped on. The smell of old milk is also pretty gross, and I would be hard pressed to find a new mom who looks forward to sleep regressions. And these are just a few of the shared experiences most postpartum moms have. These common experiences serve as an important reminder that we aren't who we were twelve weeks ago, twelve months ago . . . but that we are moms now. And our mom identity is "supposed" to be our whole identity, regardless of what came before motherhood.

When I was postpartum for the first time, I thought I wanted solutions. Sleep solutions, feeding solutions, relationship solutions, work/life balance solutions, and time management solutions. This is what I thought I needed to be the best mom, the most fulfilled in my role and the most productive in all different areas of my life. But what I eventually learned is that I didn't need solutions. I needed validation; I needed to be seen in my transition into motherhood. I needed someone to tell me that it was okay to feel lost, okay to feel like I was losing myself the deeper into motherhood I got.

And mostly I needed time to learn that postpartum would completely transform the person I had been into the person I was becoming.

My Postpartum Experience

I felt strong in my identity, and then I had a baby who loved nursing so much that my identity turned into that of a human bottle.

I came to this realization for myself after I spent three years nursing around the clock. I nursed both of my kids, my daughter for longer than I expected and way longer than I wanted to. By the time she was three, I felt like I wanted to crawl out of my skin each time she asked for "boo-boos." With the goal of weaning her, my husband went out of town with both kids in hopes that upon their return she might forget that she loved the comforts of my breasts. It didn't work. And I returned to being a bottle lady, my whole identity that of a milkmaid.

In the earliest days of my second round of postpartum, my daughter's NICU stay had turned into me overcompensating. I felt incredibly guilty that she had stayed in the hospital for three weeks after my discharge. Instead of her being home with me, taking contact naps and nursing on demand, she was fed with a feeding tube and slept alone in her hospital bassinet. And when she came home, I indulged in every single moment of skin-to-skin contact I could because I loved her and I felt bad that she had "missed out" on these connections for her first thirty days—even though I was spending six to nine hours with her every day, engaging in skin-to-skin, rocking in the NICU rocking chair.

I had lost myself in the identity of Pandemic NICU Mom With a Toddler at Home.

After three years of nursing, I was smacked in the face with the realization that so many of us live in conflict between our own ideals and the reality of early motherhood. I had spent those years pouring myself into my children, convinced that if I just gave enough of myself—my time, my body, my energy—I would somehow feel a congruency between my identity outside of motherhood and my identity within it. Because isn't that what we're told? That once you become a mother, it should be *enough*? That the deep, all-encompassing love for your child should automatically fulfill you in a way nothing else ever has?

Samantha's Story

Samantha sat across from me, her shoulders slumped, exhaustion etched into her face. "I feel like I should be happy," she said, twisting the hem of her sweatshirt between her fingers. "I *am* happy. I love my kids. I wanted this. But . . ." She let out a slow, shaky breath. "I don't love *this*—being needed every second of the day, never having a moment that belongs to just me."

I nodded, giving her space to continue.

She glanced at the ceiling as if searching for the right words. "I used to be interesting," she admitted with a quiet laugh. "I read books. I had opinions about things that had nothing to do with sleep regressions or snack schedules. I used to feel . . . like me." She sighed. "Now I feel like I'm disappearing. Like I'm *only* a mom. And the worst part? I feel guilty for even saying that out loud."

"What makes you feel guilty?" I questioned.

She hesitated. "Like I'm being ungrateful. Like if I don't *love every part* of motherhood, then maybe I'm not as good at it as I should be. I mean, isn't this supposed to be the most fulfilling thing I've ever done?"

"Who told you that?" I asked gently.

Her brow furrowed. "I . . . I don't know. It's just *out there*, right? Like, once you become a mom, that's your most important role. And it *is* important. I know that. But does it have to be *everything*?"

"That's a big question," I said. "What if motherhood isn't meant to *complete* you? What if it's meant to *expand* you?"

Her eyes widened slightly. "Expand me?"

I nodded. "What if being a mother doesn't mean erasing the person you were before but instead adding to her? What if your love for your kids and your need to feel like *yourself* aren't in competition?"

She exhaled deeply, as if something inside her had loosened. "That . . . makes sense. I guess I've been waiting to feel whole in this role. Like one day I'd just wake up and feel *completely fulfilled* by it. But maybe that's the wrong thing to expect."

I smiled. "Maybe the goal isn't to be *just* a mom. Maybe it's to be a whole person who *includes* being a mom."

She nodded slowly, the idea sinking in. "So . . . I can love my kids *and* love the things that make me feel like me?"

"Not only can you," I said, "but you *should*. You're not failing at motherhood by making space for yourself. You're showing your kids what it looks like to live a whole, meaningful life."

Samantha sat with that for a moment, then let out a small, almost relieved laugh. "I like that. I want that."

"And you deserve that," I said. "So, let's talk about what reclaiming yourself might look like—what small steps you can take to integrate motherhood into who you already are instead of letting it replace you."

For the first time in the session, Samantha sat up a little straighter. "Yeah," she said. "Let's do that."

Perfectionism sets us up to struggle more than we have to during postpartum. Perfectionism isn't such a rare quality, particularly when we're talking about women who become mothers after already having committed years to their education and career. Many of the self-identified "type A" or perfectionist moms I talk with share the same sentiment: The postpartum learning curve was brutal, and not being good at it was hard.

The Postpartum Perfectionist Audit

Many new moms feel like they're constantly falling short—but the problem isn't them. It's the unrealistic expectations they've been taught to chase. This Perfectionist Audit helps uncover hidden pressures and beliefs that might be making early motherhood harder than it needs to be. The goal isn't to become a "better" mom—it's to feel more grounded, confident, and free to mother in a way that actually works for you. How many of these feel familiar to you?

1. I anticipate the needs of everyone around me before my own.
2. I am quick to criticize myself (and sometimes my partner).

3. I believe things should be done a certain way—my way.
4. I avoid leaving my baby with others because they won't do it like I can.
5. I only feel like I've done a good job when I get the exact results I want.
6. I struggle to make decisions, even small ones.

If several of these resonate, you're not alone. Recognizing these patterns is the first step toward letting go of perfection and embracing the mother you already are.

I'm going to give you what probably feels like the worst advice ever, but hear me out:

LOWER YOUR STANDARDS. I bet you'll enjoy your identity in all areas if you allow yourself to lower the standards, if even just a little.

When I say lower your standards, what I mean is give yourself grace to grow into your new identity. Your mental health will thank you. Research shows that the impact of perfectionism can include increased anxiety, burnout, disappointment, and a lot of negative self-talk. Which would you choose: a sink full of dishes after a good nap, or functioning 24-7 without rest?

We know that becoming a mom monumentally shifts everything. But have you ever thought about early motherhood as a milestone? One that is recognized as similar to adolescence in that it reshapes our identity and our priorities in lasting and majorly profound ways?

My husband recently introduced me to the term identity saliency, which refers to the prominence of a particular identity in an individual's self-concept at any given time. It's our self-perception, how we rank our own identities at any given point. Before becoming a mom, I would have ranked my identities as such: Wife, Dog Mom, Therapist, Sister, Daughter, Friend. After becoming a mom, I would rank them this way: Mom, Wife, therapist when not momming, sister/daughter/friend when I have any time or energy left over.

During the early months and years of motherhood, the influence of our "mother" identity usually turns into the only identity we see in ourselves, or at least the biggest piece of the pie. And this can lead to a profound shift in how women see themselves, particularly if we had other strong identities—professional, partner, family member—that feel sidelined now that we're a mom.

This loss of self can feel really jarring. Women who once found pride and purpose in their careers may now struggle with feelings of inadequacy or irrelevance as they step away from professional roles. Hobbies might be abandoned, and social lives could be put on hold. A woman who thrived in a high-powered corporate job may feel alienated by the domestic focus of postpartum. Similarly, a mother who prioritized creative pursuits may feel stifled by the repetitive and mundane tasks of caregiving. These internal tensions are compounded by external pressures to "love every moment." Those of us who valued independence may feel trapped by the relentless demands of caregiving, which leave little time for pursuits that once filled our time and built our fulfillment. The intensity of this identity shift can create a vacuum where self-doubt and resentment flourish.

When I'm working with new moms who are having a difficult time with their new-mom identity, I like to explore how they can reclaim or integrate their pre-baby identities while embracing their new role as a mom. In doing so, we reframe becoming a mom not as turning into a completely different person but as achieving one's own developmental milestone.

Anthropologist Dana Raphael coined the term "Matrescence" in the 1970s. Matrescence is the process of becoming a mother.

The physical, psychological, and emotional changes you go through after the birth of your child is matrescence. When learning about matrescence myself, I found that I better understood the idea when I framed it in two different ways: first, by taking a look at how society views motherhood now, and second, by considering how would we talk about motherhood if we saw it as a milestone.

The way we think about motherhood isn't just personal—it's shaped by generations of cultural messaging, family norms, and societal pressures. For centuries, motherhood has been framed as a natural, inevitable role for women, with little room for questioning or complexity. These expectations are often so deeply ingrained that we don't even recognize them as assumptions—we just accept them as "the way things are."

Here are some of the common (and often unrealistic) ways modern culture frames motherhood:

- An expected life choice after a certain age.
- A slight change in responsibilities.
- A limited range of emotions and experiences, with the expectation that attachment and love will be prominent emotions.
- An expectation that your private life stays private and doesn't bleed into any other areas of your life.
- An identity that is *all* about the baby.

These assumptions don't just shape how we see motherhood; they also shape how we see ourselves. When reality doesn't match up with these expectations, many moms feel like they're failing. But the truth is, these beliefs were never designed to support real mothers—they were designed to uphold an impossible ideal.

Unlike the narrow, perfectionist ideals of motherhood we've been handed, the shifts in perspective listed below are rooted in what actually helps moms feel more supported, capable, and whole.

When we can acknowledge that motherhood is complex—full of change, adjustment, and emotional nuance—we create space for moms to navigate their experiences with more self-compassion and less guilt. Here's how we can reframe the transition to motherhood in a way that actually works:

- Motherhood is a developmental process that involves emotional, psychological, and physical changes that take time to adjust to.
- Motherhood is an experience of mixed emotions.
- Becoming a mother is not just about the baby but a significant change in a woman's identity.
- Motherhood is the experience of women becoming moms.

When I reframed it for myself in that way, it created two critical shifts for me. Like any significant identity shift, matrescence is supposed to be filled with emotional highs and emotional lows. Expecting constant joy not only dismisses the work of changing identity but also completely overlooks the emotional complexities of welcoming a baby. If we are going to look at motherhood as a developmental milestone, then we need to step into a space where we understand dueling emotions as a natural part of growth. And from this new lens, these are motherhood truths that I know to be true:

- Many feelings can exist at the same time. You can love your baby, and struggle to manage how quickly life changes when a baby is born.
- Motherhood is a gradual developmental change that happens over time.
- Much of motherhood is a set of learned skills.

When I launched 4th Trimester Wellness, my first ever post read "Mama, you aren't going to love every second of motherhood, and that's ok." I can tell you with certainty that the sentiment I share the most with new moms in therapy and online is that loving your baby and loving every moment of motherhood aren't mutually exclusive. Two truths can exist at once. And missing your pre-baby life, or not feeling like your new identity as mom fits you very well doesn't mean you're doing anything wrong, it doesn't mean that you're ungrateful and it surely doesn't mean that you don't love your baby.

Becoming a mother is a significant milestone, one that brings about profound changes to our identity, roles, and self-perception. It is the only time in our adult lives that we must fully renegotiate our sense of self in relation to the world around us. If we're completely honest, the truth is that much of the beginning work of becoming a mom is making magic out of the mundane. Caring for ourselves and our changing identity after having a baby is, to some, a much bigger mountain to climb than learning to care for our babies.

Jessica's Story

Jessica first came to see me for therapy when she was twenty-two weeks pregnant. She was high achieving in her career and had a partner who was supportive of her. She originally hadn't planned to be a mother, so this pregnancy was a surprise and an adjustment. She came to therapy hoping to process her pregnancy and prepare for motherhood.

We talked a lot about her family and the future family she envisioned for herself. We talked about her partner and how she didn't want to get married. We talked about her plans once the baby arrived. Throughout her pregnancy, she planned on returning to work. We met throughout the remainder of her pregnancy and also once her baby had arrived. During one of our first postpartum sessions, I stood the entire session, bouncing up and down with her baby, to give her a break. This was common; I was often handed the baby so moms could have a moment free from caregiving.

After a few postpartum sessions, Jessica asked me if she had made a mistake. She missed her life without an alarm clock, she missed feeling rested, she missed being able to buy a plane ticket on a whim, she missed the freedom and fun in her relationship. She didn't see herself as a mom. She loved her baby but didn't identify with parenthood.

And there was absolutely nothing wrong with her. She was at the very beginning of forming a new identity. She was looking for solutions to the normal challenges of early parenthood. She hadn't learned to trust herself yet, and like so many new moms, she just wanted someone to tell her what to do. She believed the myth that we must love every moment of motherhood and wasn't giving herself the permission to see becoming a mother as a developmental milestone for herself.

In her raw moments, Jessica, like many new moms, sought out all the products and recommendations, hoping they would make motherhood more manageable. Eventually, as she settled into her new rhythm—returning to work, reconnecting with parts of herself she thought she had lost—Jessica realized something crucial: She hadn't needed to change who she was to fit into motherhood. She needed to allow motherhood to grow around who she already was. It wasn't the things that made the difference; it was the care, the patience, and the permission to evolve at her own pace.

For so many new moms, the solution isn't about fixing themselves—it's about unlearning the pressure to do it all perfectly and giving themselves the space to grow into the role in their own way, in their own time.

Identity Formation During Postpartum

Before becoming a parent, many women, like Jessica, feel they have a clear sense of self built around their personal and professional lives, relationships, and passions. These aspects form the core of how we see ourselves and how we provide structure, purpose, and meaning to our lives. And then we have a baby, and everything changes very rapidly. We find our identity shifting quickly, with motherhood taking up a large portion of our time, energy, and mental space that we used to fill with different, worked-out parts of our identity. This postpartum self requires a redefining of almost everything—our priorities, responsibilities, and even our values.

In the therapy space, one of the most common conversations I have with new moms revolves around the push and pull inherent in developing a new self-concept and exploring how we identify with the different roles we play in our lives. Postpartum women often find themselves caught in a weird space of no longer relating to their life before baby and also not identifying with their new role. This tension can turn into conflict between the pre-parenting self and the post-birthing self, which then can result in all sorts of ickiness: feeling guilty for not loving every second, feeling a sense of career crisis, feeling confused in navigating all the new relationships.

Wanting to have a baby and then loving that baby doesn't change the fact that moms are suddenly faced with learning how to balance it all with who they are. On one hand, new mothers may feel immense love and dedication to their baby, but on the other hand, many express longing for the freedom, time, and energy they had before becoming a parent. This is where mom guilt is born: the intersection between our pre-life baby and our postpartum life.

Another common experience is maternal ambivalence, where we may love the moments of connection with our baby while also mourning the loss of our old routines and personal ambitions. This can also be a time of rage and high confusion. Many of the moms I have worked with describe this specific push and pull as a major challenge to navigate.

You can see this in different psychological theories of identity formation, including Erickson's theory of psychosocial development, Marcia's identity status theory, Tajfel and Turner's social identity theory, and McAdams's narrative identity theory. Psychology has spent decades studying identity development, and while these theories weren't created with postpartum in mind, they offer powerful insights into why this transition feels so disorienting—and how we can navigate it.

Identity vs. Role Confusion (Erikson's Theory of Psychosocial Development)

Erik Erikson described adolescence as the stage where we solidify our identity, a crucial developmental task where individuals explore different roles, values, and beliefs to form a cohesive sense of self. His work posits that role confusion is part of identity formation—but it also tells us that with time and exploration, we can rebuild a sense of self that integrates all parts of who we are.

What happens when you go through another major identity shift later in life? Many new moms find themselves back in a version of this struggle: *Who am I now? Do I still belong in the spaces that used to define me? How do I reconcile my past self with my present reality?*

For example, when I became a mom, I found myself questioning whether I still belonged in certain conversations. I was still the same person who loved deep discussions about books and philosophy, but now my days revolved around feeding schedules and nap battles. I worried I had lost my ability to contribute meaningfully to the world outside of my child.

Exploration and Commitment (Marcia's Identity Status Theory)

James Marcia expanded on Erikson's work by identifying four identity statuses:

1. **Identity achievement:** You've explored different roles and made a firm commitment.
2. **Moratorium:** You're actively exploring but haven't committed yet.
3. **Foreclosure:** You've made commitments without exploring other options.
4. **Identity diffusion:** You're neither exploring nor committing.

Postpartum often throws women into a state of moratorium—a period of intense exploration without a clear commitment to a new identity. Many moms say, "I don't know who I am anymore." That's because they're actively trying to reconcile old and new selves, testing out what parts of their pre-baby identity still fit and what needs to change. And that's normal. You don't have to have it all figured out right away.

Social Identity and Motherhood (Tajfel and Turner's Social Identity Theory)

Tajfel and Turner's social identity theory is founded on the idea that a person's self-concept is shaped by their membership in social groups—like work, friendship circles, and motherhood groups. Their theory suggests that we don't form our identities in isolation. But what happens when entering one group (motherhood) makes it feel like you're being pushed out of another?

Many women feel this when they step away from work or find that their nonparent friends don't relate to their new reality. The loss of a social identity can feel like a loss of self. But social identity theory reminds us that identity is fluid—we aren't just *one* thing. Just as we once integrated new roles (student, professional, partner), we can integrate motherhood *without* losing everything else that defines us.

Rewriting Your Story (McAdams's Narrative Identity Theory)

Dan McAdams proposed that identity is shaped by the stories we tell about ourselves. If you've ever thought *I used to be interesting, and now I'm just a mom*, that's a narrative you're telling yourself—but it's not the only version of your story.

What if, instead, the story became *Motherhood didn't erase me; it expanded me?*

You get to decide how this transition fits into your life story. It's not about choosing between *who you were* and *who you are now*—it's about making space for both.

Navigating the natural tension that exists between our pre-baby lives and our new motherhood will be 1,000 percent easier if we can learn to be patient with ourselves and acknowledge that the process of becoming and identifying with being a mother takes time. Practice self-compassion; allow yourself time to recognize that it's okay to feel conflicted and that ambivalence doesn't diminish your love or capabilities as a mom. Continue to practice flexibility.

What would you say if I said, "Being a mom is undoubtedly a hugely significant part of your life, and it's just one role within the larger spectrum of yourself"? This is a question I ask a lot of postpartum moms. Because the conversation around missing our pre-baby life is stigmatized and saturated with guilt, this is a good jumping-off point into our self-perception after birth.

The intersection of motherhood and womanhood is complex and layered and messy. We are learning to balance our new identity, social expectations, familial narratives, and personal narratives.

Understanding the Impact of a Changing Identity

Missing who you were before motherhood is not a sign of any sort of failure; it's a symptom of your growth. You are allowed to hold space and love for both the mother you are now and the woman you've always been.

Here is a list of some of the changes that we go through between pregnancy and postpartum. This is not an exhaustive list but a way for you to put into perspective how much change you're going through.

- The physical impact of getting pregnant, being pregnant, and then recovering from childbirth
- The emotional impact of getting pregnant, being pregnant, and being postpartum
- The relationship impact of shifts in social and relational dynamics
- The impact of adding roles to your life—motherhood on top of everything you were managing before motherhood
- The impact that motherhood has on your self-concept
- The impact that postpartum has on your time and how you experience "free time"
- The impact that pregnancy and postpartum have on your priorities

This identity shift is going to come with its own set of growing pains. And these growing pains require us to rethink the idea that motherhood is an all-or-nothing situation. By accepting that it's okay to grieve parts of your former life, you're making space for this new part to grow.

Sarah's Story

Sarah came to see me shortly after finding out she and her partner were expecting. She was in her mid-thirties and had built a strong career in graphic design. She told me many times that she loved her job, reported that a large part of her identity was tied to her creative projects, and stated that she had always had a strong sense of self.

Like many of the women I've worked with, Sarah expressed that she was nervous about becoming a mom. She made statements like "Everyone keeps telling me that I'm going to be a new person, but I like the person that I already am, and now I'm scared that everything is going to change and I'm going to lose myself in this new role as mom." She was wrestling with the idea that there would be Sarah before baby and then Sarah after baby, and the two wouldn't exist with any congruency.

Sarah and I began to work on breaking down this perspective. Instead of framing motherhood as something that would replace her current sense of self, I asked her what it would feel like to frame it as role expansion, a deepening of who she already was.

We explored looking at motherhood as the addition of a new dimension, and this perspective resonated with her. As she moved through her pregnancy, we continued to explore the traits she defined herself by—her creativity, her problem-solving skills, her ability to change course and move between tasks—and how these skills would serve her as a mother. By reframing motherhood as a new part of her existing identity, she was able to shed her idea that everything was about to change and, more importantly, that she was losing something.

This shift in perspective—allowing motherhood to be integrated into her new role—allowed Sarah to navigate becoming a mother without the pressure to be perfect or conform to some mysterious version of becoming a mom. Instead of feeling stifled, she felt like motherhood allowed her to grow, stretch, expand, and become a more layered version of her already self-assured self. We were able to work through the tensions between motherhood and womanhood and come to the understanding that one lends itself to the other, and we explored how becoming a mother isn't an 8 × 10 canvas but rather a video that keeps going.

It is completely normal to miss parts of your pre-baby life. It's completely normal to step into motherhood without identifying fully as a mom. Longing for moments of self-fulfillment—whether it's feeling you have the freedom to pursue your passions, the time to have spontaneous nights out, or the ability to spend any amount of time uninterrupted time to shower—doesn't make you bad or mean or wrong. Instead, these feelings reflect a deep, ongoing transformation of your identity. This is a natural shift, as challenging as it may feel.

Love, Marriage, and Changing Identities

The ideal of romantic love tells us that love alone will keep you and your partner connected during pregnancy and early parenthood.

"If we love each other enough, we'll figure it out."

That's what so many couples believe as they prepare for parenthood. They fantasize about the long hours they'll spend together with their new baby, imagining that they'll instinctively know how to support each other and that their deep love will be enough to carry them through the challenges of postpartum. After all, they've always been a great team; why should this be any different?

But then the baby arrives, and love alone doesn't soothe the exhaustion, miscommunication, and unspoken resentments that start creeping in. One partner feels like they're carrying the entire mental load, while the other feels like they can't do anything right. Conversations that once felt easy turn into tense exchanges about who got more sleep or who is doing "more." Moments that should feel joyful—like watching their baby smile for the first time—are clouded by an undercurrent of emotional distance.

This isn't because love isn't real. It's because the myth that "love alone is enough" sets new parents up to feel like failures when they struggle. The truth is, the postpartum period is one of the most relationship-straining times in a couple's life, and even the strongest love needs intentional support.

The idea that love should come effortlessly is a fairy tale. What actually strengthens a relationship during postpartum isn't just love—it's communication, flexibility, and a willingness to grow together.

Here are some ways to talk to your partner to strengthen your relationship during this transition:

- **Check in regularly:** Set aside time (even just ten minutes) to talk about how you're both feeling, without problem-solving or criticism.
- **Use "we" language:** Instead of "I'm doing everything," try "I feel overwhelmed—can we find a way to balance things more?"

- **Be specific about your needs:** Instead of assuming the other person knows what to do, say, "It would really help me if you handled bath time tonight."
- **Acknowledge each other's efforts:** A simple "Thank you for handling that" can go a long way.
- **Plan ahead for hard moments:** Talk about how you'll handle night wakings, household chores, and alone time before frustration builds.
- **Normalize change:** Remind each other that adjusting to parenthood is a process and that feeling disconnected at times doesn't mean your relationship is broken.

Intentional conversations like these can help prevent resentment from building and keep your connection strong as you navigate parenthood together. Remember, you're a team.

You are working toward integrating your pre-baby identity and being a mom. And with that, let's take a look at our Road Map to Change, where we'll practice different ways to integrate the dueling realities of life with a baby.

Road Map to Change: Embracing Dual Realities

This road map offers actionable steps to help you navigate postpartum identity changes with authenticity, grace, and self-compassion.

In motherhood, these are the things I experience each day at the same time, in complete opposition to each other. Maybe you can relate?

- Grateful and exhausted
- Joyful and overwhelmed
- Proud and insecure

- Connected and lonely
- Content and restless
- Confident and anxious
- Patient and incredibly impatient

The goal here is to help you navigate the complexities that exist within dueling emotions, and ultimately to accept them as okay and to love yourself regardless of how much you are loving or not loving postpartum.

Through validation, support, and self-compassion, it's possible to find joy and meaning in motherhood without denying its challenges. This road map is a starting point—a guide to navigating postpartum with authenticity and resilience, one imperfect, beautiful moment at a time.

By debunking the myth that we must *only* identify as mothers, we make space for a more honest, compassionate understanding of the postpartum experience. This myth isn't about the moments themselves; it's about the pressure to frame every moment as beautiful, regardless of how we actually feel. The truth is that the early days of motherhood are messy, exhausting, and at times overwhelming. Acknowledging this doesn't diminish the love we feel for our children—it deepens it by allowing us to embrace the reality of our shared humanity.

As we let go of the expectation to love every moment, we make room for authenticity and connection. When we recognize that our struggles don't define us as mothers, we allow grace to step and see ourselves as humans navigating a life-altering transformation. Motherhood isn't about perfection—it's about showing up, learning as you go, and finding moments of joy within the chaos—not because you're expected to, but because they're yours to hold on to.

Grab your journal or your notes app and brainstorm ways you can integrate each of these pieces into your early motherhood experience. Use the following exercises as an opportunity to reflect on how postpartum can be part of your identity in a way that allows space for you to also have an identity outside of motherhood. I ask new moms to revisit these questions and reflections throughout the first year of motherhood to stay engaged in understanding their transition.

Road Map to Change Exercises

VALIDATE THE FULL RANGE OF POSTPARTUM EXPERIENCES

One of the most liberating truths for new mothers is that it's okay to not feel completely settled into your mom identity just yet. Postpartum is a mix of joy, exhaustion, love, and frustration. Recognizing and validating this range of emotions is essential to breaking the cycle of unrealistic expectations. I recommend writing these down in a journal or recording them in your notes app as a reminder for when you're needing to normalize your feelings, create safe spaces, and challenge unrealistic expectations.

- **Normalize difficult emotions:** Acknowledge that feelings like sadness, anger, and resentment are common and don't make someone a bad mother.
- **Create safe spaces:** In parenting groups, on social media platforms, and among friends, encourage open conversations where mothers can share their experiences honestly.
- **Challenge unrealistic expectations:** Push back against societal pressures that idealize motherhood. Replace "You should love every moment" with "It's okay to feel however you feel."

Here are some reflection questions to answer now and to revisit later to see how beautifully you're evolving in your new role:

1. What emotions have surprised you the most during postpartum? Are there feelings you didn't expect to have, and how have you processed them?
2. When have you felt pressure to experience motherhood a certain way? How did those expectations align (or not) with your reality?
3. Where do you feel safest expressing your honest experiences of motherhood? If you don't have that space yet, what might help you create it?

REDEFINE SUCCESS IN MOTHERHOOD

Many mothers struggle with feelings of inadequacy when their reality doesn't match the societal ideal. Redefining what success looks like in postpartum can help mothers reclaim their confidence and joy.

- Celebrate small wins: Success doesn't have to mean a perfectly clean house or a baby who sleeps through the night. Sometimes, success is taking a shower or finding five minutes to yourself.
- Reject perfectionism: Perfectionism can trap mothers in a cycle of self-doubt and burnout. Lowering self-imposed standards is not failure; it's self-preservation.
- Focus on connection: Shift the focus from outcomes (like sleep schedules or feeding routines) to building a loving and attuned connection with your baby.

Reflection Questions

1. What small wins have you had today, even if they feel insignificant? How can you give yourself more credit for these moments?

2. In what ways has perfectionism shaped your expectations of motherhood? How can you challenge the belief that you need to "get it all right" to be a good mom?
3. How do you know when you feel most connected to your baby? What helps you focus on that connection rather than external measures of success?

RECLAIM PRE-BABY IDENTITIES

The postpartum period often feels like a time of identity upheaval. While it's natural for "mother" to become a dominant identity, it's crucial to nurture other aspects of yourself so you can feel whole.

- Reflect on your values: Take time to identify what aspects of your pre-baby self feel most important to preserve. Is it your career, hobbies, or relationships?
- Carve out time for yourself: Advocate time—even small pockets—to pursue activities that bring you joy and remind you of who you are beyond motherhood.
- Integrate your roles: Rather than viewing motherhood and other identities as competing forces, work toward integration. For example, a writer might journal about motherhood as a creative outlet.

Reflection Questions

1. What parts of your pre-baby self do you miss the most? How can you integrate those aspects into your life now, even in small ways?
2. What activities or hobbies made you feel most like yourself before becoming a mom? How can you carve out time, no matter how brief, to engage in those activities?
3. In what ways can you blend your role as a mother with other aspects of your identity? Can you think of any creative or practical ways to allow all parts of you to coexist?

BUILD AND LEAN ON SUPPORT SYSTEMS

Motherhood was never meant to be a solo endeavor, yet many mothers feel isolated and overwhelmed in postpartum. Building a supportive village can make the transition more manageable.

- **Seek emotional support:** Join postpartum groups, online communities, or therapy sessions where you can connect with others who understand your journey.
- **Delegate responsibilities:** Share caregiving duties with partners, family members, or trusted friends. Accepting help is a sign of strength, not weakness.
- **Advocate policy changes:** Support policies that provide paid parental leave, affordable childcare, and postpartum health care. Systemic changes are necessary to alleviate the burden on individual mothers.

Reflection Questions

1. Who in your life can you turn to for emotional support during this postpartum period? How can you reach out to them or invite them into your journey?
2. Are there specific responsibilities or tasks that you can delegate or share with others? How can you communicate your needs and allow others to step in without feeling guilty?
3. What policies or systemic changes would help reduce the burden on mothers? How can you support or advocate for these changes in your community or workplace?

RECOGNIZE POSTPARTUM AS A MILESTONE

The postpartum period is a profound developmental stage, akin to adolescence, where identity shifts and new priorities emerge. Viewing it as a milestone can bring perspective and compassion.

- **Acknowledge the transition:** Recognize that immediate postpartum is temporary, and also a significant phase of personal growth.
- **Honor your evolution:** Celebrate the ways you are growing and adapting, even if the process feels messy or uncomfortable.
- **Give yourself time:** Identity shifts take time to unfold. Patience with yourself is key.

Reflection Questions

1. What are the most significant changes you've noticed in yourself since becoming a mother? How have these changes shaped your perspective on life?
2. What aspects of your postpartum journey are you most proud of? Even if they feel small or messy, what growth or evolution can you honor?
3. How can you practice patience with yourself as your identity continues to shift in the postpartum period? What does giving yourself time to grow and adapt look like in your life right now?

Three Important Things

1. You are undergoing massive changes in your identity. Instead of taking care of only yourself, your pets, and your partner, you are now likely feeling the weight of caring for this tiny little person and helping them become an awesome adult person.
2. The postpartum experience is really intense, in all ways; it's okay to not love every moment.
3. Acknowledging that many feelings can exist at once will help you see feelings as fluid; remember you won't feel how you're feeling right now forever.

What's next? I will leave you with this question: If you need help, does it mean you're failing?

7

The Myth That Self-Sufficiency = Success in Postpartum

Many of us mothers arrive at postpartum with a sense of individual responsibility so deeply rooted that we dismiss any notion of needing support. We believe that requiring support reflects a lack of ability. It's as if "it takes a village" applies only to other moms—those perceived as somehow less capable. But the expectation of being able to "do it all" (care for, nurture, raise, keep a home, have a job, be a great partner, and so on) can feel incredibly burdensome. Many new mothers come to realize how deeply ingrained their standards of self-reliance and perfectionism have become only after they give birth.

The myth of self-sufficiency for new mothers perpetuates an impossible standard—the belief that a "good" mom should be able to handle everything on her own, without needing help, rest, or emotional support. This myth suggests that relying on others is a sign of weakness or failure rather than a normal and necessary part of motherhood. We've been conditioned to see the "perfect mom" as someone who handles every aspect of motherhood flawlessly and independently. But this narrative discourages us from accepting our own vulnerabilities, preventing us from building the village of support that's essential to our own survival.

I learned this lesson on my first day alone at home as a new mom. After six weeks, my mom was returning to California later that morning, and my husband was returning to work full-time after dropping my mom at the airport. I can still vividly picture myself sitting on one end of our L-shaped couch while my mom and my husband sat on the opposite side. I was hysterical, puffy faced, drenched in tears, begging them to stay with me. "You can't leave, I don't know what I'm doing, please don't leave. I'm scared to be alone; what if Jack doesn't like me?"

My husband reminded me that if I needed him, he was fifteen minutes away and would come home. He told me to call him a thousand times if I needed to, and assured me that our six-week-old loved me and that the only thing Jack didn't like was his bassinet. Which I knew to be true, but I had already decided that our baby liked my husband better.

"Honey, you can do this," my mom said. "I've been watching you do it beautifully for six weeks. If you feel trapped, go for a walk. If you feel scared, call Richie. If you need a reminder that you can do this, call me. Please make sure you're eating and drinking enough water. Jack will tell you what he needs, but you're already ten steps ahead of all his needs. I promise."

And then they left, which was painful at the time, but looking back, I'm glad they did. Because it was in their leaving that I started to build my IRL postpartum village outside of my husband and my mom. I started going on coffee dates with other new moms. I built a business and connected with new professional mentors. Their leaving forced me to reckon with myself. I had to learn that no matter how capable I felt, the transition into motherhood would require support. I needed to unlearn the assumption that self-sufficiency is the only right way. I needed a community—even just one best friend—to remember that I could do it, I was already doing it, and that this time of life is hard, in some way or another, for everyone. And this push, stepping out of my comfort zone, forced me to build my village.

What Nursing Taught Me About Self-Sufficiency

Before I had my kids, I didn't know that nursing a baby doesn't just happen. I figured I would be handed my first baby, I would put him to my breasts, he'd suckle away, and eventually, someday in the future, we'd stop nursing. Not only had I not thought about how I wanted to feed my baby, but I knew nothing about formula, bottles, nipple confusion, overnight feeding, weaning and using cabbage to dry out milk supply and fenugreek to make more of it.

I left the hospital with our son and a plan in place, a plan that I didn't really agree to but instead fell into. I would triple feed him: put baby to breast, then pump, then bottle feed until he was content. I was supposed to be nursing him every two to three hours, and this whole triple-feeding process took about an hour at minimum, so by the time I was done it was time to start over, and I didn't have the stamina to continue triple feeding for too long. Within two weeks of being postpartum, I developed both oversupply and several rounds of mastitis.

I had such an oversupply that I started dripping breast milk when I was only sixteen weeks into my second pregnancy. Enough milk for the whole village. I would joke that in a past life I must have been a milkmaid. Jokes aside, during the earliest days of postpartum I was in constant pain from both the weight of my breasts and the pressure of keeping twenty to fifty ounces of milk on board at any given time.

Early in my first postpartum, my breasts began to look like orange peels—which can be a sign of a particular form of breast cancer. After a ton of back-and-forth and sending nip pics via the online portal with my midwives, it was recommended that I undergo testing at the breast cancer center to make sure that I didn't have breast cancer. This all happened within the first four weeks of parenting. It was terrifying. I felt out of my depth in terms of my ability to cope with the shift into postpartum and the thought of having breast cancer with a new baby.

The physicians ran their tests and then came back to tell me that everything was okay and referred me to the hospital's outpatient lactation consultant and feeding group for new moms. This is where I met Karen, the nurse and lactation consultant who became my daytime breast wizard village.

For me, following through with the referral was a double challenge—not only was I a first-time mom, but I was also a perfectionist who had relied so heavily on self-sufficiency that those around me always assumed I could handle any situation without help. I had no idea how to hand express, I had no idea what mastitis was, and I had no idea what a lactation group was. I had set the expectation of complete self-sufficiency in every area of my life, and now I was learning that there was no place for perfection—either for myself or for my family—in my new role as a first-time mom.

Karen and I had two or three one-on-one consultations where she watched and supported my son and me in our nursing extravaganza, and she invited me to join the feeding group as Jack and I continued to work on breastfeeding. I loved her; I still love her. I was probably one of hundreds, if not thousands, of postpartum moms she has worked with over the years, and I felt cared for and supported and educated.

When my mom left and my husband returned to work, Karen became the first part of my postpartum village. I wasn't going to be able to do this alone. My identity was different now, and I needed to be surrounded by and supported by people who understood that a woman isn't the same after having a baby. I didn't realize how meaningful the support Karen had offered me was until I ran into her at work many, many months later—and was still nursing my son successfully.

Modern moms are sent two very distinct and very opposing messages about being a mom. The first: It takes a village. The second: You should be able to do and want to do all of the early parenting on your own. Want the help, but don't take the help.

Have a village, but don't rely on your village. This personal experience was not an isolated one but rather what I've come to identify as a reflection of a larger societal shift that has slowly redefined the foundation of parenting support.

Lauren's Story

When Lauren walked into my office, she looked exhausted. Not just tired—exhausted in a way that had settled deep into her bones. She collapsed onto the couch with a sigh, adjusting the baby strapped to her chest.

"I don't know what's wrong with me," she said, shaking her head. "I love my baby, but I feel like I'm failing. Everyone else seems to handle this stage so much better. My mom raised four kids without help. My grandmother had six. Why can't I do this with just one?"

I let her words settle in the space between us before gently asking, "Where did you get the idea that you should be able to do this alone?"

She blinked at me, as if the question had caught her off guard. "Isn't that just . . . what moms do?" she said hesitantly. "I mean, I'm on maternity leave. My husband helps when he can, but he works long hours. My mom keeps telling me that this is just what new mothers go through, that I need to get through it. That she managed, so I should too."

Her voice broke on the last words, and she looked away, embarrassed.

"I just thought I'd be better at this," she admitted.

I nodded, recognizing the weight of her words. "Lauren, let me ask you something. When your mom was raising you, do you think she truly did it all on her own?"

She frowned. "I mean, she had my dad. And my grandmother lived nearby. And the neighbors . . . they all kind of helped each other out."

I smiled. "That sounds like a village."

Lauren was quiet for a moment, staring down at her sleeping baby.

"I guess I just don't have that," she said softly.

"Not yet," I said. "But that doesn't mean you can't build it."

We spent the rest of the session unpacking her belief that "good moms" do it all alone and where that idea had come from. We talked about how independence is often mistaken for strength when in reality strength comes from knowing when to lean on others. I asked her what support would actually feel helpful right now—not just what she thought she was supposed to handle alone.

By the end of the session, Lauren wasn't magically "fixed"—because this isn't about fixing. But she left with something just as powerful: permission. Permission to reach out. Permission to ask for help. Permission to redefine what it meant to be a good mother—not as someone who did it all alone but as someone who recognized that motherhood was never meant to be a solo endeavor.

And that is where the healing begins.

Understanding the Stories We've Absorbed

In the United States, if you deliver in a hospital or birthing center, you are sent home shortly after having a baby. Which seems obvious but doesn't hit home for most new moms until they're home alone without support staff, nurses, lactation consultants. Some of us may have a family that comes and stays for a short bit to help, and then, for partnered couples, one usually returns to work and the other is home with the baby managing most of the infant care. For me, this highlights just how much Americans hold to the ideal of self-sufficiency and the individualistic approach that we take into, well, everything we do.

In the US, postpartum doulas and home visits are considered a luxury limited to those with financial resources, while in other areas of the world, it is common practice for midwives or other health care workers to provide home visits during the earliest days of postpartum. In Mexico and some other Latin American countries, there is a period after childbirth called la cuarentena, a practice that stems from the belief that after the vaginal canal is opened for the baby's birth, the woman is also reborn and needs time to rest, recover, and return to vitality. At the end of the forty-day practice, the mom receives a hot bath to finish cleaning the uterus and mark the end of the gestational period. Forty days, or six weeks, postpartum is around the time that the uterus has returned to its prepregnancy size.

In the Netherlands, whether you give birth at home or in a hospital, a trained professional called a kraamverzorgster visits the home daily for eight to ten days following birth. They provide medical checks for birthing parents and the baby. They can also help other children in the family acclimate to life with a new baby. Their services are generally covered by insurance, and if it isn't covered by insurance, they are available at a low cost.

In Nigeria, *omugwo* is the Igbo word used for the postpartum caregiving that a mother provides for her daughter or daughter-in-law following birth. Different tribes have different names for similar practices where nourishment and rest are the key focus.

For centuries, extended families formed the foundation of community organization, providing collective support for raising a baby, resource sharing, and caregiving. In agrarian communities, it was common for multiple generations to live together, sharing all responsibilities in ways that blended individual roles with community needs. Postpartum moms had access to a wide network of support people who were all invested in the well-being and upbringing of the new baby.

This collective approach distributed the physical demands of parenting and allowed for emotional, psychological, and physical support for new moms. The concept of "it takes a village to raise a child" was not an aspiration, it was an understanding and a lived reality. Within communal systems, the responsibilities of parenting weren't left for the mom; they were shared as a value of family and community.

The shift to a nuclear family model began in the early nineteenth century and accelerated during the Industrial Revolution. Urbanization, the rise of wage labor, and the economic pressures of industrialization encouraged families to move further away from extended family networks, and this migration toward cities reshaped the ways families could support each other. In response, family units began to narrow, eventually becoming parents and kids in a home away from other family. While this shift provided some opportunities for autonomy and mobility, it also introduced new pressures, particularly on mothers, to manage the house and childcare without external support.

The nuclear family became the dominant model in the mid-twentieth century, particularly in Western societies. Post–World War II economic growth, suburbanization, and the influence of media solidified this new family structure as aspirational: a home in the suburbs, dad working outside of the house, and mom at home raising babies and managing the household. The nuclear family—made up of a breadwinning father, a stay-at-home mother, and their children—was glorified as the pinnacle of progress and familial stability.

This twisted ideal was heavily propagated through advertising, television, and political rhetoric. Families began to see women as domestic caretakers who effortlessly managed their homes and children with little external support in popular media. These portrayals ignored the complexities of what parenting looks like and set a new precedent: Being a good mom meant being a perfect mom, and it was the mom's job to be entirely self-reliant within the confines of a beautiful suburban home.

The cultural evolution of the nuclear family supported a narrative that motherhood was a marker of competence and worth. This is the moment in history when we cemented the notion that relying on extended family, friends, and community meant a mom was failing to fulfill her role. When families started moving into suburban sprawl, the toll of isolation began to manifest, and some moms began to identify their loneliness and dissatisfaction.

The rise of the nuclear family reshaped parenting and supported the myth of self-sufficiency. This rigid division of labor, with mothers staying home and fathers working outside the home, was presented as the natural order, but it left mothers with little autonomy and fewer opportunities to seek support outside of their immediate household.

Fast-forward to today, where culturally we've changed—many women work outside the home and dual-income households are the norm—but the expectation that mothers should shoulder the bulk of childcare persists. The infrastructure to support working parents, such as affordable childcare and paid parental leave, remains inadequate, especially in the United States. This creates a "double shift" for mothers who often carry the majority of the domestic labor and caregiving responsibilities before and after their work hours. The myth of self-sufficiency—rooted in the 1950s ideal—continues to pressure moms to "do it all," despite the vastly different demands of modern life.

Today, new mothers are often left to navigate the complexities of parenthood in relative isolation. The proliferation of social media has only exacerbated this issue by perpetuating unrealistic standards of perfection. This supermom myth—rooted in the self-sufficient homemaker ideal of the 1950s—has evolved into a pressure cooker of expectations, with moms feeling compelled to excel in parenting, career, socially, all while projecting an image of effortless success.

The Myth of Self-Sufficiency in My Family

I am a millennial mom. I had my first baby at thirty-three and my second at thirty-six. My mom is a boomer mom. She had her first baby at twenty-seven and her second at thirty. My grandma Doris was part of the Greatest Generation. She was thirty when she had her first child, thirty-two when she had her second, and thirty-seven when she had her third child. The ideal of self-sufficiency in womanhood and in motherhood looked different for each of us, but it has remained unchanged in its demands. This expectation to be a "strong mom" and a "capable woman" is the thread that's woven us together, outside of being family, even outside of being mothers.

For my grandma Doris, self-sufficiency was born out of necessity. As a child she experienced the trauma of illness, leading to long periods of isolation. She worked to provide financial assistance to her parents and lived at home until she was married at twenty-eight. Her self-sufficiency in her young adult life into her married life was part of fulfilling the unspoken obligations of her time and place. As she aged into her marriage and into motherhood, she held her family together quietly, gracefully, and with little assertion of her own needs. Her role was a role of duty—providing love and care within the boundaries of traditional gender roles, a deep unconditional love, and an unspoken understanding of what a good wife and mother should be.

My mom, as a boomer mom, embraced a different kind of self-sufficiency. She became a mom living away from her own parents, her friends, and much of her community. Like her own mom, my mom carried the weight of domestic duties and carried them mainly on her own. Self-sufficiency for her generation meant proving she could juggle everything—running her own business, being a mom, and taking care of a household—while my dad devoted himself to building his career and career successes. It was a balancing act steeped in a desire for validation, connection, and care.

And when I became a mom, the expectation of self-sufficiency had evolved but remained just as unrelenting. In many ways, I was better equipped. I had more education and more access to resources. I began parenting in a time where unsolicited parenting advice was everywhere, from books to blogs to social media. But the core expectation of being able to do it all and figure it all out remained unchanged.

If anything, this expectation for modern moms has intensified. Unlike my mom or grandma, I am expected not only to raise my children and maintain a career but also to prioritize my career, my self-care, and my individuality outside of my roles of mom and wife. I feel lucky to be raising kids at the time I'm raising kids but also see our generation of moms as the generation who has been told we can have it all without being told *how* we can have and manage it all. Modern motherhood demands that we thrive in all areas, for many moms without a village to lean on.

My fellow therapist mom friends have joked about how quickly we dismissed support during our own postpartum experiences, responding "No, I'm good," or "No, I've got this," because that's what we figured was expected of us. Yet the irony is that each generation of mothers in my family has been, in some way, deeply dependent. My grandma relied on her neighbors. My mom leaned on her neighbors. And I rely on my mom and my mother-in-law and my friends. And still, we all mostly mothered alone. The expectation of self-sufficiency in motherhood is almost more exhausting than actual motherhood.

If I could talk to my grandma now, I'd want to ask her how she felt about the expectations placed on her as a mother and wife. Did she like being married? Did she like keeping a home? Was it what she wanted? Did she want something more? What I do know is that her quiet and steady care were her legacy, passed down to my mom and then to my sister and me. And that maybe it's time to let go of the expectation that mothers should be silent martyrs or endlessly capable superwomen. Instead, maybe we could embrace a new generational thread: the courage to admit we don't have it all figured out, the support to ask for help, and the grace to know that's more than enough.

From Self-Sufficient to True Support

From the moment a baby is born, new mothers are bombarded with the expectation that they can integrate their pre-baby life with their post-baby life seamlessly and with little support. This gives me the ick. Is there much of motherhood that I can do alone? Yes. But should I? Absolutely not.

Beyond the mental health impacts of isolation and redefining what help can look like, the economic realities of modern motherhood make complete self-sufficiency nearly impossible. In the United States, where paid parental leave is not a guarantee, many moms are returning to work within weeks of giving birth. This lack of systemic support places an additional burden on moms. While postpartum doulas, lactation consultants, and therapists can provide valuable support, these services are expensive and not inaccessible for many families. On the same note, outsourcing support is limited to those who can afford it.

The day-to-day reality of life with a new baby is both profound and overwhelming. One of the most common themes that I hear from new moms is that they are lonely. Loneliness has a profound impact on our mental health, affecting us emotionally, cognitively, and physically. Chronic loneliness—persistent feelings of being socially or emotionally disconnected (hello, postpartum)—can have lasting impacts on our confidence, sense of community, and mental health.

We have a loneliness epidemic among new parents, and the ideal of self-sufficiency has created a wave of moms who don't even have enough support to focus on their physical recovery from childbirth, let alone sensory overload and the learning curve of becoming a mom.

Loneliness can contribute to:

- Persistent sadness, loss of interest in activities you once enjoyed, and difficulty finding meaning in your day-to-day life
- Fear of rejection, feelings that you don't belong, increased worry, increased stress responses, hypervigilance, or becoming overly sensitive to perceived social cues
- Impaired cognitive function over time, including worsened short-term and working memory
- Reduced self-esteem, leaving you feeling unworthy and leading to further withdrawal, inadequacy, and shame
- Increased risk of substance use to numb big feelings

Ironically enough, loneliness can be a self-feeding cycle. When we are feeling lonely, we can in turn avoid social interactions out of fear of rejection or awkwardness. This withdrawal can reinforce feelings of isolation, making it harder and harder to break the cycle.

Most new moms have been inundated with messages that glorify independence—doing it all without asking for help, taking on every night shift, every day shift, and doing it without complaint. While consumerism might tell us this is empowering, it often leaves new moms feeling more isolated, overwhelmed, and unsupported during a critical time of adjustment and growth.

Postpartum care has looked very different across different cultures. Whereas communal care used to be the gold standard of postpartum, allowing the community to help so the mom can rest and recover, this isn't the reality for many parents anymore. The nuclear family structure of the 1950s has morphed into geographical dispersion from extended family, meaning many new parents are having to find other means of support.

I believe that the way help is conceptualized during the postpartum period needs a fundamental overhaul. A new mom shouldn't feel ashamed of asking for help or exist inside cultural conditioning that equates needing help with inadequacy. As a result of this conditioning, we often reject offers of support that don't align with our perception of what help should look like—often it's framed as help with the baby rather than help for the mother herself.

This needs to change. Help during the postpartum period isn't just about holding the baby while the mom showers or takes a nap. It's also about emotional support, helping out with older siblings or pets, and providing a nonjudgmental space for processing the seismic identity shifts that accompany motherhood.

To redefine postpartum support, we need to shift the focus from asking moms what they can do for everyone else to asking what can be done for them. A few practical examples include:

- **Flexible social support.** Instead of vague offers like "Let me know if you need anything," friends and family should focus on making specific, actionable offers—for example, "I'm going to the grocery store today. I'm going to drop dinner off at the door and will text you!" or "What day can I come do your laundry?"
- **Professional resources.** Increasing access to doula support, lactation support, and mental health supports can help level the playing field for new families that don't have extra income to spend on such services.
- **Building community.** Encouraging mothers to connect with others through new-mom groups, local parenting organizations, or online forums can alleviate feelings of loneliness and foster more of a shared experience.

- **Partner involvement.** Equipping partners with education so they can participate fully in parenting and household responsibilities can help redistribute the emotional and physical workload. This also helps partners jump in and not feel on the outside of life between baby and mom.
- **Workplace and policy changes.** Paid parental leave and more accommodating work environments are essential for families to thrive. Advocating systemic changes that support mothers and their families is critical for long-term progress.

In addition to external support, there's an emotional and psychological shift that needs to take place for mothers to embrace help. Asking for help isn't a sign of weakness or failure; rather, it's an act of strength and self-awareness. Reframing the postpartum period as a time of collective effort rather than solitary endurance can help dismantle the stigma around receiving help.

The reframing also involves educating new moms about the unrealistic expectations set by societal norms. Motherhood is not about performing a role perfectly but about navigating a deeply imperfect transition. Accepting help will never diminish your role—it will only help enrich it by allowing you to prioritize your recovery and your transition.

And for those of you thinking *I don't want a village. I don't want people in my home. I can't imagine trying to sit in a coffee shop with a three-week-old baby*—I hear you. Like, I totally hear you. Truly. Postpartum is an incredibly vulnerable time, and the thought of opening up our space or life to others can feel overwhelming, even intrusive.

For many of us, the idea of having a village isn't something that feels practical or even appealing. You wait until you're ready, and if you never feel ready, eventually your kids will be making friends and you'll meet the parents. They still don't have to be your village, but one of them could end up being your later-in-life bestie.

And if you fall into this camp, I'll offer you this: Your village doesn't have to look like whatever you're dreading. It doesn't have to involve people you aren't comfortable with. It doesn't have to mean hosting, or even having people in your home. Your village can be whatever you feel supports you the best, even if that is simply letting your partner completely take over bath time and bedtime for your baby so you can get some alone time. Your partner—they're your village too.

The point is, help comes in many different forms, and it doesn't have to disrupt your comfort or boundaries. You can design your version of your village—one that meets your needs and feels safe, manageable, and supportive. Accepting help doesn't mean inviting chaos into your home; it means giving yourself permission to be cared for, even in ways that feel small.

When you begin to think about your village, start small. What's one thing that would make your day just a little easier? Who's one person you could trust to show up in a way that feels right for you? Building a village doesn't happen overnight, and it doesn't have to look like anyone else's. It's about creating space for connection on your terms, in ways that honor both your needs and your boundaries.

The myth of the self-sufficient mother is just that—a fallacy. Human beings are inherently social beings; we are wired for connection and collaboration. Parenthood is no exception. It is time we move away from the outdated notion of solitary maternal efforts and toward a model of shared responsibilities.

The road map forward lies in celebrating interdependence: fostering a culture where asking for and offering help is normalized and valued. Interdependence recognizes that thriving as a mother, partner, and individual is a collective effort, not a solo performance. By shifting the narrative from "doing it all" to "doing it together," we can create a postpartum experience that honors the needs of both mother and baby while also cultivating stronger communities. This is not just about surviving postpartum—it's about redefining it as a time of profound growth that includes healing and connection.

Road Map to Change: Learning to Celebrate Interdependence

Moving away from the myth of self-sufficient motherhood requires small, intentional steps that help redefine support and community. These steps encourage you to embrace interdependence—a model that values connection, collaboration, and raising a child as a shared responsibility.

Remember, you are parenting in a different time in history. Be quick with transparency and communicate your needs. Also remember to always assume the best intentions.

By taking these steps, you move closer to a model of parenting that prioritizes authenticity, connection, and well-being. Interdependence isn't about giving up your autonomy or identity, it's about weaving together new threads of support that allow everyone to thrive. It's about valuing collaboration over isolation and learning to celebrate the beauty of shared efforts.

Redefining help during the postpartum period is a radical act of self-care and community building. When we embrace interdependence, we honor the truth that motherhood was never meant to be a solo endeavor but a shared journey that makes all of us better and allows us to more fully love.

Postpartum can feel like a test of endurance, and the myth that a mom is only doing it "right" if they're doing it all and doing it alone doesn't help anyone. This myth thrives on the idea of self-reliance as a measure of success in parenting, when really embracing a postpartum village is not just an option, it's necessary for sustainability.

Here's the good news: The postpartum village doesn't have to look like a scene from a party. It can be built intentionally, piece by piece, to reflect your values and your needs. It can include virtual support, doulas, friends, family. It doesn't matter who makes up your village; what matters is that you're not doing it alone.

Imagine a world where mothers feel empowered to say, "I can't do this alone, and I'm not supposed to." Imagine a world where every new mom is surrounded by a village that uplifts her, whether that's through a neighbor dropping off a meal, a friend watching the baby so she can nap, or a text thread of fellow moms reminding her she's not alone. That's the world we need to build.

The postpartum village isn't a relic of the past—it's a lifeline for the present and the future. Embracing it doesn't make you less of a mother; it makes you a more resilient, supported, and connected one. Let's stop perpetuating the myth that motherhood is a solitary journey. Instead, let's reclaim the village and remind every mom that she was never meant to do this alone.

Now that we've explored why asking for help is not a sign of weakness but an essential part of thriving in postpartum, let's talk about *how* to actually do it. It's one thing to recognize the importance of support but another to actively build and lean on a village. The following steps offer practical ways to reframe asking for help, create a strong support system, and normalize shared responsibilities. These are not just theoretical ideas—they are actionable strategies you can start using today to feel less overwhelmed and more connected.

Road Map to Change Exercises

Each of these sections includes simple, intentional ways to build your network, share responsibilities, and shift your mindset around help. You don't have to implement them all at once—start small and see what feels right for you.

REFRAME ASKING FOR HELP

Begin to think of asking for help as a gift to both yourself and your baby. Frame support as an opportunity for connection rather than a sign you are doing something wrong.

For example, instead of *I don't want to burden them by asking for help*, try *They want to support me, and I could use some one-on-one time with another adult; what a gift to have this option.*

Ideas on how to start:

- Make a list of tasks or areas where support would be helpful. Put the list on your refrigerator and use it as a reference when someone wants to help you.
- Practice asking for help with a small task from a trusted friend or family member. Like saying yes when someone offers to bring you coffee, or stop by and go for a walk.

BUILDING YOUR HELP MAP

This looks like creating a network of support that includes friends, family, and professionals.

Ideas on how to start:

- Make a list of people or resources who could help in different areas—emotional support, household tasks, baby care, etc.
- Include professionals like lactation consultants, postpartum care professionals, and therapists in your plan.
- Share the map with your partner (it's better even if you create the map together) and make a plan for when it's time to activate!

NORMALIZE SHARED RESPONSIBILITIES

This looks like communicating openly about the division of labor at home.

Ideas on how to start:

- Hold a conversation with your partner or your household members about shared parenting and household tasks.
- Instead of assigning roles, use a collaborative approach: "What do we feel we can each take on?"
- Check in weekly to redistribute responsibilities as needed.

CONNECT WITH YOUR VILLAGE

This looks like actively seeking out or creating a community of support.

Ideas on how to start:

- Join local or online mom groups—walking stroller group, new-mom book club, mommy-and-me yoga.
- Seek out groups that are specific to postpartum moms so you can find other moms in the same stage of motherhood.
- Host a "mommy coffee hour" at your house with friends and neighbors.

REDEFINE THE IDEA OF PERFECT HELP

If we wait for perfect help, we could be waiting a really, really long time.

Ideas on how to start:

- If someone you trust offers to help, accept the help, even if it's not exactly how you want something done. For example, your sister-in-law comes over and asks if she can fold the laundry—let her. Even if it isn't how you would do it, let her do it and check it off of your list.
- To piggyback on that idea, work on practicing gratitude for the intention behind the help rather than focusing on the execution.

LEARN TO SAY YES AND NO STRATEGICALLY

This looks like protecting your energy by balancing when to accept and decline offers of help or social obligations.

Ideas on how to start:

- Work on saying yes to offers that align with your needs. "Yes, I would love help with grocery shopping." "I would love if you could pick up Pepper at doggy day care."
- Say no without guilt to anything that feels draining or unnecessary. You're allowed to say no.

EMBRACE INTERGENERATIONAL SUPPORT

This looks like learning to include family members in your postpartum. For some, this might be cousins; for others, it's great-aunts. If you have family around you, reconnect!

Ideas on how to start:

- Get curious about the parenting stories of your grandparents or older relatives. Ask them to share their experiences and begin building understanding and building connections.
- Delegate tasks that play to their strengths. My mom is a great cuddler, and my MIL is a great teacher. Our kids get the best of both worlds.
- Set clear expectations about your parenting style to avoid misunderstandings.

Three Important Things

1. Being able to manage everything on your own is not a measure of success. Asking for help also isn't a measure of success. Doing what you need for your own well-being—that is a measure of growth.
2. *You get to decide what support looks like.* There isn't a right or wrong way to open yourself up to support; you find the way that works best for you.
3. Postpartum support is a means of self-care. One more time: Receiving support during any period of parenting is self-care.

What's coming next? I leave you with this question: How have you been treating your postpartum body?

8

The Myth of the Perfect Postpartum Body

After Jack was born, I lost the "baby weight" plus an additional twenty-ish pounds within the first six weeks postpartum. I was praised for how great I looked, how amazingly my body had bounced back, and I was encouraged to keep doing whatever I was doing. What I was doing was having panic attacks. I spent four to six weeks not being able to eat because my anxiety was so bad.

My rapid postpartum weight loss was the first time I had been confronted, personally, with the expectation of thinness—and I wasn't even skinny; I was just smaller than I had been prepregnancy. As someone who's always had a more mature figure, I had never dealt with weight loss praise. And it felt really, really fucked up. I was being praised for having a baby and not looking like I had just had a baby.

The myth of the postpartum bounce-back is one of the main culprits in perpetuating the harmful expectation that new mothers should strive to quickly return to their prepregnancy bodies, prioritizing appearance over health and recovery.

It's a curious phenomenon that happens when a baby is born: While we're still in the fog of sleepless nights, healing bodies, and changing hormones, the world seems to collectively lean in, look at mom, and say things like, "How much weight did you gain?" "Have you started exercising yet?" "I have great weight loss tips whenever you want them!" Whether people speak blatantly or more subtly, we can thank a culture that glorifies quick fixes, snapback bodies, and a return to "normal" for why the pressure to lose weight exists. It's a myth so normalized that it's rarely questioned. But it should be.

The idea of "bouncing back" implies that pregnancy is a phase you should endure and emerge from unchanged, both physically and mentally. But this expectation ignores the reality that pregnancy and childbirth change you, deeply and permanently. It reshapes your body, rewires your brain, and shifts almost everything in your life. To suggest otherwise is to deny the profound transformation of bringing a new life into the world.

This myth isn't just about unrealistic beauty standards, though those play a significant role. It's about a broader societal discomfort with change and an insistence that women's lives, ambitions, and appearances remain untouched by the monumental experience of motherhood. The pressure to "bounce back" doesn't just set mothers up for failure; it undermines the beauty and value of the postpartum period.

The "Bounce-Back" Myth

Pregnancy changes our bodies, *and* it's supposed to. Before I had my first kid, I knew close to nothing about what actually happens to our bodies when we're pregnant. I just listened to the apps that told me how big my baby was, equivalent to whatever the fruit of the week was. I didn't know what a sciatic nerve was, I didn't know what relaxin was, I didn't know what colostrum was. I learned, sort of, but mostly I just watched my body change and assumed it was all normal. So for the sake of actually understanding our bodies and how massively they adapt the moment we get pregnant, let's have a little anatomy lesson.

From the moment of conception, hormones begin to take over. Progesterone is the first overachiever, as it begins relaxing the muscles in your uterus to keep the baby in its place. But this isn't the only place that it relaxes. Progesterone also relaxes your digestive tract (hello, heartburn!). Add in estrogen for your pregnancy glow; hCG, which gives you your positive pregnancy test; and relaxin, which softens your ligaments. You have now become a full cocktail of new hormone surges.

In the meantime, your uterus has a major growth spurt, starting out as the size of a pear and growing to accommodate a baby the size of a watermelon. This means that your organs have moved aside. Your bladder becomes a pancake, your lungs lose their space, and your skin begins to stretch.

You may see stretch marks on your belly, hips, breasts, or thighs. This is your body actually stretching to make room for your growing baby. Some of us are blessed with a radiant glow thanks to increased blood flow and oil production, while others get teenage breakouts. Either way, our skin becomes a visual diary of the changes that are happening in us.

Then there's our heart, which is working overtime to support the growth and health of our baby. Our blood volume increases by up to 50 percent, which is essential for our baby but less ideal for our veins, which may bulge into varicose veins. Swelling in our feet and hands, courtesy of fluid retention, becomes another companion. If you can see your feet by the end of your pregnancy, you may barely recognize them. My feet grew a whole size during my pregnancies.

Our breasts also embark on their own transformation, preparing to feed a baby. Tenderness and growth are early signs, and by the third trimester, some of us (this was me) may notice colostrum leaking. They are another tangible reminder that our bodies are undergoing an epic change.

Our digestive system slows due to hormones, leading to our favorite pregnancy symptoms: heartburn, constipation, and morning sickness. Pelvic floor muscles stretch to support our growing uterus as we prepare for childbirth. These muscles endure immense pressure. Everything on the inside is *changing*, and changing fast.

Understanding these changes matters, because when we talk about postpartum bounce-back, we're talking about an unrealistic expectation that our bodies will magically erase nine months of effort overnight. If we expect our bodies to look or feel a certain way, it's crucial to grasp the enormity of the changes they just went through. The truth is these transformations are a testament to our body's resilience and adaptability. We should be celebrating our body's hard work, not actively working to make sure there is no trace of having been pregnant.

And then we have a baby and a body that just grew a baby, and that takes time to recover from. Generally, postpartum recovery happens in stages, from immediate postpartum to longer-term adjustments that can take years.

Immediately after childbirth, the uterus begins a process of contracting to return to its prepregnancy size. This process is facilitated by oxytocin, which is the culprit for cramping and afterpains, especially during breastfeeding. The vagina and the perineum, particularly for women who experience tears or an episiotomy, begin to heal, which can take weeks to months, depending on the severity of the tissue damage and the amount of scar tissue that develops. The lochia, or vaginal discharge that consists of blood, mucus, and uterine tissue, results from the uterus shedding its lining and can persist for up to six weeks. If you're a C-section mama, you too will have this discharge.

Our pelvic floor muscles often require additional attention that we don't give them during our postpartum recovery. It's common for women to experience weakness in these muscles. Think of your pelvic floor this way: It's a big basket that holds everything in and together when we're pregnant. It has to work really, really hard under a whole lot of pressure. Pelvic floor physical therapy has emerged as an effective intervention to restore strength and function to revitalize these muscles.

Feeding our baby also introduces additional physical demands. While we know the benefits of breastfeeding, we talk less about sore nipples, engorgement, and clogged ducts. In some cases, me being the case four different times, we can face mastitis, which comes with an additional set of medical needs.

Postpartum recovery is also different for moms who experience cesarean deliveries, birthing trauma, adoption, birth of multiples, premature birth, infant loss, and a whole array of birthing situations outside of a traditional vaginal birth. Body image is a significant factor in how we navigate our postpartum lives. If you get dressed and feel icky, are in pain, or are focused on the sizes that fit, you are more likely to cancel plans, talk negatively to yourself, and isolate yourself.

And as societal beauty standards continue to dominate our focus, we risk falling into cycles of thinking there's something wrong with us. Why didn't our bodies bounce back like those of the celebrities who are celebrated for losing their baby weight four minutes after having a baby? While comments like "Look at how strong you are" may acknowledge our resilience, they don't always resonate when we don't like the way we look.

Sam's Story

Sam arrived at our first session and was very direct. "I hate my body," she said. "It took me years to love my body, and then I got pregnant, and then I had a baby, and now I'm back to hating my body. And I'm incredibly touched out and overstimulated. Basically, I feel like I'm crawling out of my skin all of the time."

She told me about a history of struggles with food and body image. She didn't speak of any history of disordered eating, but she did talk about her own mom, who was obsessed with the way both of them looked and was immediately already buying her daughter the gaudiest of outfits. Sam retraced a long family history of pressure to look a certain way, regardless of the circumstances (going through puberty, early college). During our first few meetings, Sam wasn't quite able to separate the expectations that her mom had for her with the expectations she had for herself.

As our sessions continued, Sam began to unpack the generational messaging she had received about appearance and self-worth. She described how her mother's constant emphasis on weight and presentation had shaped her own sense of value. "She was always dieting," Sam said, "and she always made comments—about herself, about me, even about strangers. I grew up thinking that being thin wasn't just important; it was everything."

During our conversations, we explored how these ingrained beliefs were colliding with her postpartum experience. She felt trapped between a social expectation to "bounce back" and her body's reality after carrying and delivering a baby. "I want to love my body, I want to be able to see myself as strong, but all I see is fat."

One of our early goals was to help Sam distinguish between the voices of external expectations—her mother's, society's—and her own inner voice. This process took time. At the beginning, when I asked Sam what she wanted for herself, she struggled to answer. "I don't even know," she shared. "I've spent so much time worrying about what other people think."

Using a few different tools, we began to create space for Sam's own thoughts and desires. She found she loved guided journaling, and after each session I would create a list of questions for her. Each week, the last question was always "How did you make yourself proud this week?" Over the weeks, Sam's list of ways she was making herself proud grew. She was overcoming breastfeeding challenges and saying yes to plans, and slowly her lists started to include ways she was proud of her body. She started to include things like maintaining her daily stroller walk, focusing on her hydration, and listening to how her body felt versus what size she was fitting into that week.

In our body image work, we also addressed the experience of feeling touched out, as she often found herself feeling overstimulated and irritable at the end of the day. We did a lot of processing around sensory overwhelm in postpartum life, and we worked on developing practical strategies. Whether it was accepting support or time blocking her day, she started to identify little rituals that she could use to slow everything down.

After working on identifying her values, what she wanted, and how she felt, we started to work on setting boundaries with her mom—gently but firmly. Sam began to understand that her mom's feelings didn't have to be her truth; they also didn't have to be her feelings. Sam also started to understand that while she wouldn't be able to change her mom, she could change how she approached her mom.

Slowly but surely Sam began to start healing the part of her that had been attached to the validation and feedback from those around her. She started to identify the type of mom she wanted to be and the role that body image was going to play in parenting her own daughter. In one of our final sessions, Sam was reflective. She had come to see our work not as a race to return to her pre-baby self but as an opportunity to grow into a new, more self-loving person grounded in strength and self-compassion. She had worked really hard and had arrived at a place of giving herself permission to just be.

The Ideal of Thinness

Inhale, exhale. Are you ready? Let's talk about the ideal of thinness, skinny as a sign of perfection, health, beauty, success, and all things bounce-back.

We live in a time where skinny privilege is real. The social, cultural, and systemic advantages that people in thinner bodies experience compared to those in larger bodies are everywhere we look. These privileges exist because of established societal norms and biases that value thinness and stigmatize fatness, often in ways that are deeply ingrained and generally go unquestioned. While this doesn't mean that thin people don't face challenges, it highlights the ways in which they are less likely to encounter specific forms of discrimination or marginalization that people in larger bodies routinely face.

Skinny privilege significantly impacts pregnant people, as it impacts how women are treated in health care settings and in social spaces and touches on broader cultural narratives about pregnancy. For those in thinner or smaller bodies, societal biases often work to their advantage, whereas individuals in larger bodies are more likely to face heightened stigma, discrimination, and negative assumptions that affect their pregnancy experience.

Pregnant people in thinner bodies are less likely to have their health concerns dismissed or attributed solely to their weight. In contrast, people in larger bodies are more likely to encounter fatphobia in regard to getting pregnant and experiencing complications. Larger-bodied pregnant people are assumed to be less healthy, regardless of their actual health status. Every pregnant person should be treated as an individual and provided care as such.

Just as we have medicalized the birthing process, we have medicalized and pathologized "fatness." We've bought into the idea that fatness is always inherently abnormal, undesirable, or dangerous, and any blanket statement that stigmatizes larger bodies is awful for a postpartum mom. Or any mom. Or any woman. Really, it's awful for all of us.

Historically, fatness has not always been stigmatized. In many ancient cultures, larger bodies symbolized wealth, fertility, and health—particularly in times and places where food scarcity was common.

The Venus figurines dating from 28,000 to 20,000 BCE are some of the most iconic representations of pregnancy and fertility, and these figures emphasized features such as large breasts, wide hips, and rounded bellies as symbols of fertility and abundance and the ability to sustain life.

It wasn't until the eighteenth and nineteenth centuries, with the growth of modern medicine, that being large began to be classified as a medical condition. This shift marked the beginning of fatness being viewed through a pathological lens. Fast-forward to today, and the contrast between ancient ideals of a bountiful postpartum body and modern body standards becomes even more pronounced.

The history of and development of the body mass index—or BMI—further cemented the medicalization of our body size, and it is extremely problematic. BMI was created by Adolphe Quetelet, who was . . . wait for it . . . an astronomer, mathematician, statistician and sociologist. Originally, BMI was never intended to measure individual health but was used as a tool for studying population statistics.

BMI has been criticized for being flawed and an overly simplistic measure of health, as its inception was part of Quetelet's work to define the "average man" in European populations. So when BMI was widely adopted in the twentieth century as a health metric, it continued to reflect the body types and health norms of white European populations. And this Eurocentric foundation ignored the biological, cultural, and lifestyle differences that exist across other racial and ethnic groups, making BMI an inherently narrow and exclusionary standard.

BMI enforces a universal standard of "ideal" body weight that does not consider cultural or historical diversity in what constitutes health and wellness. With time, body size became a reflection of new American values—if you are fat, you lack discipline, efficiency, and the ability to be productive, and the size of your body is a matter of morality more than genetics. So while BMI is often used as a quick and easy health metric, its origins and application are deeply flawed.

Our cultural obsession with thinness, particularly in the context of pregnancy and postpartum, perpetuates unattainable ideals that then create additional pressure for new parents navigating the physical and emotional demands of childbearing. Pregnancy, once celebrated for its transformative power and connection to life, is now often scrutinized through the lens of aesthetics, with an emphasis on bouncing back or maintaining a certain body image throughout the perinatal period.

This fixation on thinness doesn't just impact how new moms feel about themselves—it can also affect how willing women are to seek care before, during, and after their pregnancy. Larger-bodied individuals may face dismissive attitudes from health care providers, excessive monitoring during pregnancy, or unnecessary interventions, all rooted in assumptions that are made based on a person's size. This disparity illustrates how deep the biases about body size can be in perpetuating harmful stereotypes.

The implications extend beyond pregnancy into postpartum life, where new parents are inundated with messages about "getting your body back"—a phrase loaded with the insinuation that their own postpartum body is bad. This rhetoric erases the profound physical and emotional labor of childbirth, reducing a life-altering experience to a simplistic and harmful beauty standard. For larger-bodied postpartum parents, these pressures are often compounded by a societal fear of being larger, which in turn can make postpartum lonelier or isolating.

The historical context of body ideals reminds us that these standards are not fixed truths but instead cultural constructs that evolve over time. When we can recognize this, we can help challenge the harmful narratives surrounding body size, pregnancy, and motherhood. It's crucial to move toward a more inclusive and compassionate approach that honors the diversity of our bodies and experiences.

Pregnant Bodies Through the Ages

Body standards and beauty in pregnancy have evolved with time and across cultures. Let's take a look:

- **40,000–10,000 BCE:** The Venus figurines—Venus of Willendorf (Austria), Venus of Hohle Fels (Germany), and Venus of Dolní Věstonice (Czech Republic)—are small prehistoric statues of women, believed to represent fertility, womanhood, and motherhood. The figurines are full bodied, with large breasts, bellies, and hips.
- **Ancient Greece (800 BCE–146 BCE):** Think goddesses like Hera. Full-bodied, curvaceous figures represented health, motherhood, and divinity. Pregnant bodies were celebrated as a sacred part of life.
- **Renaissance era (fourteenth–seventeenth centuries):** Artist Peter Paul Rubens's paintings elevated fuller, curvier women as the epitome of beauty and fertility. A pregnant body was a sign of wealth and power.
- **Victorian times (1837–1901)**: This is when pregnancy went undercover. Corsets and layers of clothing kept baby bumps discreet, and women were expected to hide any evidence of motherhood in public.
- **Mid-twentieth century:** Here we enter the age of the modest mom. Pregnancy became a private, sanitized experience, and moms-to-be were encouraged to regain their pre-baby bodies ASAP.
- **Today:** We're in an odd mix of bump flaunting and relentless pressure to bounce back after birth. Thinness still dominates beauty ideals, but more voices are rising to embrace body diversity.

The next time you're feeling pressure about your postpartum body, remember beauty standards have changed dramatically over the centuries and they'll change again. But even more importantly, you get to define beauty for yourself.

Body Positivity: Good and Bad for Postpartum

The body-positive movement has been instrumental in challenging the "bounce-back" culture that pressures moms to quickly return to their prepregnancy bodies. By celebrating postpartum bodies in all their diverse forms, the movement validates the natural changes that come with pregnancy and childbirth, helping moms feel less alone and less pressured to cave to unrealistic ideals.

Representation in social media campaigns and public discourse has also played a key role. Images that include stretch marks, loose skin, and postpartum curves have made many moms feel seen and valued, fostering self-compassion and pride in what their bodies have accomplished.

However, the body-positive movement isn't without its drawbacks for new moms. One of the challenges lies in the pressure to feel positive about your body all the time. While the movement emphasizes self-love, this expectation can make moms feel inadequate or guilty if they struggle with their postpartum appearance or the physical changes they've undergone. And some aspects of the movement oversimplify complex feelings about postpartum bodies, offering messages like "Just love yourself!" that can feel dismissive to those grappling with their body image after pregnancy. Social media, though a powerful tool for representation, can also exacerbate this issue. Even the "real" portrayals of postpartum bodies are often curated and idealized, making self-acceptance seem effortless and unattainable for many.

Additionally, the movement's focus on appearance, even in its effort to decenter traditional beauty standards, can inadvertently reinforce the idea that a mom's value is tied to how her body looks. This emphasis can overshadow more pressing postpartum concerns, such as mental health, sleep deprivation, and the identity shifts that come with motherhood. For new moms, striking a balance between appreciating their bodies and navigating the broader challenges is crucial.

Ultimately, while the body-positive movement has made significant strides in validating and celebrating postpartum bodies, it needs to be complemented by messages that embrace the full range of the postpartum experience. New moms benefit most from a culture that not only normalizes the natural changes in their bodies but also supports their physical, emotional, and mental well-being without oversimplification or undue pressure.

In recent years, a growing number of organizations and movements have emerged to challenge harmful beauty standards and promote body acceptance—particularly for new mothers navigating the physical and emotional shifts of postpartum. Among them, groups like The Body Positive, Be Nourished, and Health At Every Size (HAES) have been instrumental in reframing how we think about health, self-love, and body neutrality.

For postpartum moms, these organizations provide a crucial counterpoint to the relentless pressure to "bounce back." They offer resources, community support, and advocacy aimed at helping women reconnect with their bodies on their own terms—whether that means learning to appreciate their postpartum form, focusing on function over appearance, or simply letting go of external expectations altogether.

As we well know at this point, correlation does not equal causation. Many of the studies linking weight and poor health fail to account for confounding variables, such as socioeconomic status, access to health care, weight stigma, and chronic dieting. In fact, weight cycling—or repeatedly losing and regaining weight—has been shown to have significant negative health effects, including increased inflammation, higher blood pressure, and greater risk of cardiovascular disease.

Weight stigma has far-reaching consequences for both our physical and mental health. In what world did it become okay to tell someone "Just lose weight" instead of working to understand the underlying concerns of the patient? At its heart, body neutrality is about equity. It challenges the systemic biases that prioritize thin bodies and marginalize those in larger ones. This includes addressing the intersection of weight stigma with other forms of discrimination, such as racism, sexism, and ableism. By advocating weight inclusivity and respectful care, we can align ourselves with broader movements and pushes for a world where everyone has access to the resources and support they need to thrive.

When we're talking about postpartum specifically, hating the body we are in can have far-reaching and damaging effects in many areas of our life, from mental and physical health to relationships and the quality of the postpartum experience. Even though many of the standards we hold stem from internalized pressures and a lifetime of seeing unrealistic beauty standards, they can perpetuate a cycle of negative self-perception that is difficult to break.

Hating our body is strongly linked to mental health struggles, including depression, anxiety, and lower self-esteem. When someone constantly criticizes or feels ashamed of their body, they may experience persistent feelings of inadequacy and worthlessness. This can lead to chronic stress, chasing the ideal of "perfect," and in the most extreme cases, disordered eating.

Not loving how you look can also lead to harmful behaviors aimed at achieving a perceived ideal. Crash dieting, overexercising, or turning to weight loss medications can take a toll. On the other end of that spectrum, feeling uncomfortable in our own skin can also lead to avoidance of certain activities from feeling self-conscious about the way we look.

For postpartum individuals, body hatred can hinder our ability to embrace the changes brought naturally by pregnancy.

I often find that the most insidious impact of not liking our bodies is how it erodes our ability to practice self-compassion. When a new mom views her body as inherently flawed, it can be challenging to extend kindness or understanding to ourselves. This lack of compassion can hinder personal growth, resilience, confidence, and our ability to treat ourselves with compassion and grace. You made a baby! This doesn't deserve punishment; it deserves honoring your body's ability to adapt.

I find solace in embracing recovery, whether physical or emotional. Embracing recovery offers new moms an invaluable opportunity to heal and celebrate the resilience and adaptability of the human body, the human spirit, and the strength of women. Recovery isn't just about returning to a prepregnancy state; it's a transformative practice that allows us to witness our body's remarkable capacity to repair, rebuild, and adapt. Viewing recovery through this lens shifts the narrative from one of limitation to one of awe and gratitude.

Our bodies are designed to heal, and they initiate the intricate processes of restoring our balance and function on their own. Recovery is also a testament to our innate intelligence and how well we are able to endure. Recognizing this inherent resilience can cultivate a sense of wonder and respect for our own selves, even if we don't fit into what society deems right.

Postpartum recovery is also a time to redefine our expectations and a time we can give ourselves the permission to rest and focus inward. In a culture that glorifies productivity and perfection, slowing down and embracing your truest self is in itself an act of activism, agency, and self-determination. When we celebrate recovery, we affirm that rest is productive and that taking time to heal is not only necessary but also a deeply compassionate act of caring for ourselves.

Embracing recovery means learning to be patient and kind to yourself. Just as our bodies adapt, so do our minds. By reframing recovery as a celebration of our body's ability to adapt rather than a race to return to a previous state, we create space for pride in the process.

We never return to the version of ourselves that we were prior to having a baby. And instead of aspiring for a great return, what would happen if we embraced ourselves as we are right now and learned to love this version as full, complete, and exactly as it should be? We don't have to aspire to some vague social ideal; we have to love ourselves from the inside out and give our children the same opportunity.

Road Map to Change: Learning to Accept Your Postpartum Body

Your body has just done something extraordinary—it has grown, birthed, and nourished a human. Loving your postpartum body isn't about forcing positivity; it's about building a relationship with yourself rooted in respect, care, and appreciation.

If your efforts are rooted in self-compassion, self-expression, and your own sense of well-being, then they are always worth pursuing. But if they're driven by fear, stigma, or the idea of being othered, you deserve more. Your postpartum experience shouldn't be about your body erasing any sign of pregnancy.

Road Map to Change Exercises

LOVING YOUR POSTPARTUM BODY

Postpartum body acceptance doesn't happen overnight—it's a process of shifting your mindset and practicing self-compassion.

This activity is designed to help you reframe how you see your postpartum body, challenge unrealistic expectations, and find small ways to care for yourself.

Read through each step, try the suggested action, and take a moment to reflect. There are no right or wrong answers—just gentle ways to reconnect with and appreciate the body that has carried you through this transformation. Here are six simple steps to loving your postpartum body in a way that is rooted in self-compassion.

1. **Shift the narrative:** Instead of seeing your postpartum body as something that needs to be fixed, reframe it as a body that has evolved.

Try this: Replace critical thoughts with compassionate ones. Instead of "I miss my old body," try "My body has changed because I did something powerful."

Reflection: What is one thing your body has done in postpartum that you can appreciate today?

2. **Prioritize comfort over comparison:** Postpartum bodies are not meant to look like prepregnancy bodies. Avoid the trap of comparison—whether to your past self, celebrities, or filtered social media images.

Try this: Unfollow accounts that make you feel bad about your body. Instead, seek out body-positive postpartum content that feels real and encouraging.

Reflection: Where are you feeling the most pressure to "bounce back"? How can you challenge that expectation?

3. **Nourish, don't punish:** Your body needs fuel and care, not restriction or guilt. Focus on gentle nutrition and movement that support your energy rather than trying to "erase" the changes.

Try this: Instead of dieting, practice intuitive eating—listening to your body's hunger cues and giving it what it needs without judgment.

Reflection: What's one way you can nourish yourself today without guilt?

4. **Reconnect with your body through small acts of care:** You don't have to love every change, but you can show kindness to your body in small ways that make you feel good.

Try this: Wear clothes that fit and feel good. Take a warm bath. Moisturize your skin with care. Move in ways that bring you joy.

Reflection: What is one small act of kindness you can show your body today?

5. **Expand your definition of beauty:** Postpartum beauty is soft, strong, capable, and ever-changing.

Try this: Take photos that capture the real, unfiltered moments of motherhood—your baby asleep on your chest, your hands cradling tiny feet, your eyes filled with love.

Reflection: What is something beautiful about your body *right now*?

6. **Give yourself time:** Postpartum is a transition, and body acceptance is a process. You are allowed to take time to adjust to this new version of yourself.

Try this: When you catch yourself thinking negatively about your body, pause and ask yourself *Would I talk to a friend this way?* Then speak to yourself the same way you would speak to someone else.

Reflection: What's one way you can be patient with your body's healing today?

Your body tells the story of how you became a mother. And that's a story worth embracing.

Three Important Things

- You get to create your own beauty standards.
- You get to determine your value and worth.
- You are worthy of recovery. Your body and your baby are worthy of the time and patience it takes to recover from pregnancy and birth. Give yourself that gift.

And what's coming next? Do you understand the differences between the baby blues and perinatal mental health concerns?

9

The Myth of the Perfect Postpartum Mood

Postpartum is a time of profound joy, but it's also a time of intense emotional, physical, and psychological change. It's a time of sleepless nights, overwhelming new demands, and an identity shift so profound it can feel like the ground has been pulled out from under you. It's really no wonder that many moms experience waves of anxiety, sadness, irritability, or even rage. And yet too often we brush these feelings off as fleeting without considering that they might be signs of something other than the learning curve of new motherhood—that they may instead be symptoms of a perinatal mental health disorder.

When we talk about perinatal mental health, we're not just talking about postpartum depression (though that's certainly part of it). We're talking about a spectrum of experiences, including postpartum anxiety, postpartum obsessive-compulsive disorder, postpartum post-traumatic stress disorders, and postpartum psychosis. We're talking about the baby blues, sure, but also the full range of emotions that come with adjusting to parenthood. The myth of perfect postpartum mental health is one of the most insidious lies new mothers are fed. The image of the glowing, grateful mother basking in the warm haze of new motherhood is everywhere—in commercials, on Instagram, in the way well-meaning friends and family ask *Aren't you just loving every minute?*

This chapter is for the moms who wonder if they're the only ones struggling, who fear that their distress makes them unfit to parent, or who have bought into the myth that the postpartum period is supposed to be a time of nothing but joy and gratitude.

When we talk about postpartum mood disorders, perinatal mental health, and female reproductive health, I like to encourage new moms and moms-to-be to explore the space between their mental health and their whole identity. If you are experiencing a mental health struggle during postpartum, it isn't who you are, it's what you are experiencing. We don't need to drown ourselves with shame for existing.

Margot's Story

For Margot, this distinction became a lifeline.

In the early weeks after her daughter was born, Margot found herself gripped by an anxiety she hadn't anticipated. Every small decision felt impossibly high-stakes. She would lie awake at night, convinced that if she didn't check her baby's breathing one more time, something terrible would happen. When she did sleep, she'd jolt awake at the smallest sound, her heart racing. During the day, she worried constantly—was the baby eating enough? Was she holding her the right way? Should she be enjoying this more?

What scared Margot the most wasn't just the thoughts—it was what they meant about her as a mother. Was she failing? Was she broken? The more she spiraled, the more she began to tell herself *I'm an anxious mother. I'm not good at this.*

It wasn't until a conversation with her therapist that she began to shift her thinking. "You're not an anxious mother," her therapist said gently. "You are *experiencing* anxiety. And that's different."

That small reframing opened a door for Margot. It allowed her to see that postpartum anxiety wasn't a personal failing—it was something happening to her, not something that defined her. She began to talk about it more openly with her partner, to name the worries when they came instead of letting them consume her. Slowly, she built a tool kit: grounding exercises when the panic crept in, deep breaths before responding to an anxious thought, and, perhaps most importantly, the ability to remind herself *I am not my anxiety. I am a mother experiencing something hard, and I am getting through it.*

This shift—from *I am* to *I am experiencing*—is a powerful one. It creates space for compassion, for support, for healing. For new moms like Margot, it can be the difference between drowning in postpartum anxiety and finding a way to rise above it.

This distinction isn't just about language; it's about how we see ourselves. When we blur the line between who we *are* and what we're *going through*, it's easy to become consumed by a single identity or struggle. But by recognizing that experiences—both joyful and challenging—are just that, *experiences*, we allow ourselves the freedom to change, adapt, and seek support. This is especially important in the postpartum period, when identity itself can feel like it's shifting beneath our feet.

As we talked about in Chapter 6, we tend to rank our personal identities—for example, I'm a mom, then a wife, then a sister, daughter, friend, therapist, consultant, author . . . and so on. The line between *I am* and *I am experiencing* can be very thin. But *I am a mom* and *I am experiencing motherhood* are very different things. *I am postpartum* and *I am experiencing postpartum depression* are also very different things.

Intrusive Thoughts

When Laura came to see me, her baby was just two months old. Tears streamed down her face as she shared that she was having frequent intrusive thoughts about driving off the road with her baby in the car. She didn't have an urge to act on her thoughts, but the thoughts alone were scaring her.

I met Stacy for the first time when her baby was six months old. Shortly after meeting me, she confessed that she imagined drowning her baby during bath time—not because she wanted to, but because the image would intrude on her thoughts without warning. She was terrified and didn't know what to make of these thoughts that seemed to have come out of nowhere.

Nora came to me when her baby was four months old. She described how she couldn't stop picturing her baby being run over by a car, a horrifying thought that she couldn't shake, no matter how much she tried.

And then there was Jemma, three weeks postpartum. She admitted she was plagued by thoughts of dying in an accident and leaving her baby motherless. These thoughts weren't just fleeting, they were persistent, distressing, and completely at odds with how deeply she loved her baby.

Can we pause for a moment to honor the courage it took for these moms to say any of these words out loud? It's hard enough to experience intrusive thoughts like these—thoughts so deeply unsettling they make you question your own sanity—but to share them with another person? To open yourself up to judgment, misunderstanding, or fear? That's bravery on a whole new level.

And yet each of these women believed that their thoughts meant something terrible about them. Each one worried that saying these things out loud would result in their baby being taken away. Each one asked me some version of the same heartbreaking question: "Are you going to call Child Protective Services?" "Will I lose my baby?"

Intrusive thoughts do not make you a bad mom. The Maternal Mental Health Leadership Alliance reports that up to 70 to 100 percent of postpartum women experience unwanted or intrusive thoughts. That's right, up to 100 percent. So if you've had these thoughts too, you're not alone. And these thoughts? They don't mean there's something fundamentally wrong with you. And they don't mean that you're an unfit parent.

What they do mean is that you're going through one of the most demanding transitions of your life. Instead of looking at intrusive thoughts as threatening, try to see them as a reflection of how much you care. They're typically the worst-case scenarios that your brain conjures up in an effort to protect your baby. They're distressing, yes, but they're also a sign of just how deeply you're invested in your baby's safety and well-being.

Struggling with perinatal mental health doesn't mean you're crazy or broken. It means you're navigating an enormous amount of change, and you deserve compassion, understanding, and support.

Let's Talk About Intrusive Thoughts

Since having a baby, have you experienced unwelcome thoughts about:

- Your death?
- Your baby's death?
- You or your baby being involved in a catastrophic incident?

More importantly, have these thoughts triggered shame, embarrassment, or the feeling that you're failing because of the question *What type of mom has these thoughts?* If your answer is yes, you are not alone.

Intrusive thoughts are actually protective; they are an indicator that you are stepping into the role of caregiver, mother, nurturer, and protector. You just had a baby—and part of becoming a parent is learning to protect our babies from harm. These thoughts are a natural, normal reaction.

When confronted with unwanted postpartum thoughts, I challenge you to ask yourself the following questions (this is a great time to pull out your notes app or your journal if you want to answer now). These questions can help you shift your mental attitude toward self-compassion and acknowledge and validate your feelings without getting stuck in repetitive doom loops.

1. **Is this thought based on fact or fear?** Try to determine whether the thought is rooted in evidence or if it stems from anxiety, self-doubt, or exhaustion. For example, the fear of death does not reflect the reality that you are dying—and having anxiety about what might happen in the future doesn't actually mean that what you're fearing will happen. Most intrusive thoughts are, therefore, not based in fact.
2. **What would I say if someone else told me they were having intrusive thoughts?** By imagining how you'd comfort someone in the same situation, you may begin to be able to offer yourself the same compassion.
3. **What is the bigger picture at this moment?** Take a step back and consider how this thought fits into the larger context of postpartum. Is this type of thought fleeting or a recurring challenge?
4. **What is positive in this moment?** Even when we have unwanted thoughts, finding a glimmer in a challenging moment is a small way to shift our focus away from fear.
5. **What does my body need right now?** Unwanted thoughts could be tied to physical or emotional needs like rest, nourishment, or connection. Try to identify what might help soothe the thought or give you some relief. What I've found works really well for many of

my postpartum clients is keeping a note in their phone of positive affirmations to counter anxious or intrusive thoughts.

If you were to come into my office and have a panic attack, I would help you move through that anxiety with a grounding practice. I've included that practice here so you can try it at home yourself as well.

Grounding Practice

1. Place one hand on your heart and the other on your belly. Before looking at any of your intrusive thoughts, take five to ten very deep, grounding breaths.
2. Identify or write out what your intrusive thoughts are—for example, *I feel stuck, nothing is ever going to change, and I am stuck in the permanency of newborn life and sleep deprivation*. It can be really hard to comprehend what triggers these thoughts, especially when we're sleep deprived, so for this moment, the cause doesn't matter—we start by working on getting through the moment.
3. After writing down your thoughts, counter each of them with an alternative based in fact. For example:
   Thought: *I am stuck, and this is never going to get easier.*
   Counterthought: *I know that nothing lasts forever. Right now I am safe and supported.*
4. Take as much time as you need to regulate your nervous system.

It is so easy—I know from firsthand experience—to get carried away in cycles of obsessive or worrisome thoughts. And it is also common that once we've worked ourselves through the thought, our bodies remain in a constant state of hypervigilance. This is where learning how to physically regulate is just as important as cognitively regulating.

Understanding Perinatal Mental Health Disorders

When we understand the difference between the word *postpartum*, which refers to a period of time, and *postpartum depression*, which is a specific mental health condition, we gain clarity. When we learn about the symptoms of postpartum OCD, we can educate our loved ones about what to look for. When we normalize conversations about intrusive thoughts, we make it easier for moms to seek help without fear of judgment or shame. The stigma around postpartum mood disorders is a heavy burden, especially for moms who are already holding themselves to impossible standards of perfection. These moms feel like they're supposed to have it all together, and when they don't, shame creeps in, screaming to them that they're failing. But here's the thing: Struggling with your mental health doesn't mean you're failing. It means you're human.

So let's dive in. Let's unpack the landscape of perinatal mood disorders. Let's normalize the conversation and arm you with the knowledge and compassion you need to feel confident and comfortable in your own skin. We'll start by talking about what perinatal mental health disorders are. We'll work through the misconceptions, the signs, the symptoms, the history, and the treatment options. Because, well, you deserve to feel like yourself again. You deserve to enjoy motherhood—not as a picture-perfect ideal, but as the beautiful, challenging, and deeply human experience it is.

So take a deep breath. You've got this. And we're going to walk through it together.

From a medical standpoint, there are several stages of postpartum. The *acute postpartum* stage is characterized by rapid change with the potential for immediate crises, including postpartum hemorrhage, uterine inversion, amniotic fluid embolism, and eclampsia. Part of the reason that nurses visit the mom's room so often in the first twenty-four hours after birth is to check for signs or symptoms of any of these immediate crises. During the *subacute postpartum* stage, your body is still going through major changes in terms of blood flow, organ recovery, metabolism, and emotional well-being. These changes are less rapid than in the acute postpartum phase, and you are likely able to self-identify your concerns. The *delayed postpartum* stage is when estrogen and progesterone levels begin to return to prepregnancy levels, and this is a common time for prolactin (nursing hormones) to drop.

An important part of understanding postpartum mood disorders is understanding, generally, the hormonal changes that your body undergoes in the first three months of postpartum. Regardless of the type of birth and delivery, your hormones are going to fluctuate during these first three months. The changes in hormones can lead to mood challenges, hair shedding, and postpartum insomnia. Also, the night sweats. The "baby blues" refers to the first two weeks of postpartum, when your hormones are undergoing drastic changes.

Nearly 80 percent of new mothers will experience the baby blues in the first few weeks of postpartum. This is in response to hormonal shifts, sleep deprivation, and the learning curve of caring for a newborn. The symptoms of the baby blues could include:

- Mood swings
- Increased tearfulness
- Fatigue
- Feelings of overwhelm

The baby blues typically resolve within two weeks without treatment. However, if these feelings persist or worsen or if you become unable to manage your daily tasks, this is where it would be beneficial to be assessed for a perinatal mood disorder. Unlike the baby blues, perinatal mood and anxiety disorders (PMADs) are clinical conditions that require attention and treatment. PMADs include:

- Postpartum Depression (PPD)
- Postpartum Anxiety (PPA)
- Postpartum Obsessive-Compulsive Disorder (PPOCD)
- Postpartum Post-Traumatic Stress Disorder (PPTSD)
- Postpartum Bipolar Disorder
- Postpartum Psychosis
- Perinatal Grief and Loss-Related Disorders

Of these, postpartum Depression is the most well-known, and the most common PMAD, and includes the symptoms of:

- Persistent sadness or low mood
- Loss of interest in activities you once looked forward to
- Ongoing fatigue or lack of energy
- Noticeable changes in appetite or sleep patterns
- Feelings of worthlessness, guilt or hopelessness
- Difficulty bonding with your baby

Postpartum Depression can look like: you are able to care for your baby but can't find the energy to shower or eat. You feel a constant heaviness in your chest and you find yourself wondering if your baby would be better off without you, and then following that thought, you get filled with guilt. You are feeling unenthused and indifferent.

Postpartum depression can begin anytime within the first year of postpartum, though it will often appear within the first three months. Regardless of your history or family history of depression, PPD can affect anyone. The treatments for postpartum depression include therapy, medication management, peer support and lifestyle adjustments.

While postpartum depression garners much of the attention, postpartum anxiety is equally common. It is characterized by excessive worry and fear and an interruption of your daily functioning. The signs of postpartum anxiety include:

- Consistent worry about your or baby's health and safety
- Racing thoughts or inability to relax
- Physical symptoms like racing heart, nausea or dizziness
- Noticeable insomnia
- Avoidance of certain activities or situations out of fear

Postpartum anxiety can be accompanied by intrusive thoughts. Treatment for postpartum anxiety includes therapy, medication management, mindfulness skill building, education and therapy.

Postpartum Anxiety can look like: checking the baby every few minutes convinced that something might be wrong, despite that baby is resting peacefully. You get fixated on SIDS and have difficulty relaxing. You have a hard time putting the baby monitor down and at times have fallen asleep next to them in case of an emergency.

Postpartum Obsessive-Compulsive Disorder of Postpartum OCD is an often-overlooked PMAD but deserves attention due to its unique and distressing nature. It's marked by intrusive thoughts and compulsive behaviors aimed at neutralizing those thoughts. Signs and symptoms include:

- Intrusive thoughts about harming the baby (dropping the baby or suffocating them)
- Compulsive behaviors to prevent harm (repeatedly checking if the baby is breathing)
- Hypervigilance around the baby's safety

- Awareness that the thoughts are irrational, which distinguishes postpartum OCD from postpartum psychosis

Postpartum OCD can look like: you have waves of panic during mundane daily tasks worrying about the worst-case scenario. You experience intrusive thoughts about every accident under the sun and have a difficult time focusing.

The evidence-based treatments for postpartum OCD are cognitive behavioral therapy, medication management and education.

Postpartum Post-Traumatic Stress Disorder is often triggered by a traumatic birth experience, such as an emergency c-section, excessive medical intervention, or feeling of loss of control during labor and delivery. It is also more common for moms that have experienced trauma. Signs of postpartum PTSD can be:

- Flashbacks or nightmares about the traumatic event
- Hypervigilance or feeling constantly on edge
- Avoidance of anything that reminds you of your birth
- Emotional numbness or detachment
- Difficulty bonding with the baby due to unresolved trauma

Postpartum PTSD can look like: you have a difficult time making it through the day due to flashbacks, or nightmares, you avoid the place that the event took place (for example, the hospital) and are overcome with overwhelming fear.

The evidence-based treatments for postpartum PTSD include trauma-focused therapy modalities like EMDR or eye movement desensitization and reprocessing, support groups and medication management.

Postpartum Bipolar Disorder is a mood disorder that can occur after childbirth, characterized by extreme mood swings that range from manic or hypomanic episodes to depressive episodes. Unlike the typical mood fluctuations many women experience in the postpartum period, postpartum bipolar disorder is more intense and can significantly affect a mother's ability to care for herself or her baby. Signs of postpartum bipolar disorder can include:

- Manic or hypomanic episodes where one experiences increased energy, racing thoughts, impulsivity, feeling unusually high or overly happy, lack of need for sleep, or engaging in risky behavior.
- Depressive episodes include feelings of sadness, hopelessness, irritability, difficulty concentrating, and thoughts of self-harm or harming the baby.
- Rapid mood swings that alternate between feelings of high energy and deep depression, often within short periods of time.
- Severe mood instability or feeling "out of control" emotionally, swinging from periods of excessive energy to deep fatigue or sadness.

Evidence-based treatments for postpartum bipolar disorder include mood stabilizing medications, antidepressants, and psychotherapy. Early intervention and support from a healthcare provider specializing in perinatal mental health can help manage symptoms and improve outcomes for both the mother and her baby.

Postpartum psychosis is a rare but serious postpartum experience. It affects approximately 1-2 in every 1,000 mothers. It typically develops within the first two weeks of postpartum and requires immediate medical attention. Unlike other PMADS, postpartum psychosis can include delusions or hallucinations and poses a significant risk to both mother and baby if untreated. Signs and symptoms of postpartum psychosis include:

- Hallucinations or delusions (hearing voices that others can't hear)

- Extreme mood swings
- Confusion or disorientation
- Paranoia or irrational beliefs
- Thoughts of harming oneself or others

Postpartum Psychosis can look like: you are checking the baby's breath every five minutes and are convinced something terrible will happen. You avoid going outside, you are unable to sleep and are hearing voices that you aren't sure are real.

Postpartum psychosis is a medical emergency, and the person experiencing postpartum psychosis may not know that they are in a medical crisis. If you or someone you know is experiencing these symptoms, it is paramount to seek immediate medical attention. Evidence-based treatments of postpartum psychosis include hospitalization, medication management and therapy once stabilized.

Perinatal Grief and Loss Related Disorders refer to the emotional and psychological challenges that arise after the loss of a pregnancy, stillbirth, or infant death during the perinatal period (before, during, or shortly after birth). Grief during this time can be especially complex, as it is often accompanied by feelings of deep sorrow, guilt, and confusion, compounded by hormonal changes and the physical recovery process. Signs of perinatal grief and loss related disorders can include:

- Intense sadness or sorrow, a pervasive sense of loss, often accompanied by crying, sadness, or feelings of emptiness.
- Guilt or self-blame, questioning what you could have done differently, even though the loss was beyond your control.
- Difficulty bonding with future pregnancies or children.
- Intrusive thoughts or flashbacks
- Withdrawal from others due to feelings of inadequacy or discomfort around others.

- Physical symptoms of grief include fatigue, loss of appetite, sleep disturbances, or feelings of numbness or detachment from reality.

Perinatal grief and loss disorders can deeply impact a mother's emotional well-being, making it difficult to adjust to daily life or connect with others. It can also disrupt one's relationship with their partner, as both individuals may grieve in different ways and need different kinds of support.

Evidence-based treatments for perinatal grief and loss related disorders include grief-focused therapy, complicated grief therapy, support groups specifically for those who have experienced perinatal loss, and mindfulness-based therapies to help manage symptoms of anxiety and depression. Medication may also be considered if there are accompanying symptoms of depression or anxiety that interfere with the mother's functioning. Early intervention and professional support are vital to help mothers process their grief and find ways to cope with their loss.

Untreated PMADs can have lasting effects on the whole family system, and it is important to connect with qualified medical professionals for both a diagnosis and treatment. It is important to meet with a medical provider to discuss all treatment options.

I am often asked if there is a way to know if you will experience a perinatal mood disorder, and what can be done during pregnancy to avoid it. As annoying as this answer is, it just depends. Perinatal mood disorders can affect anyone, but certain risk factors may increase the likelihood of developing them. Some of the most prominent predispositions are having a personal or family history of mental health disorders, a history of trauma, lack of social supports or difficult interpersonal relationships, physical and medical factors, and the pressure to be perfect.

Questions to Ask Your Provider

If you are concerned about a postpartum mood disorder, here are some questions you can bring to your medical provider.

1. I have a history of ______, and I want to make sure that I have mental health support in place. What is your protocol should I need additional support?
2. Do you have a list of psychiatrists or therapists that work specifically with expectant and postpartum parents? If not, where do you suggest I find providers trained in perinatal mental health?
3. If I happen to need immediate support with my mental health, what are the resources I should have?
4. I am planning on breastfeeding, can you provide me with education on what medications are safe to use while breastfeeding?
5. After my baby is born, who do I resume medical care with?

There are many resources available to you, and I highly recommend finding postpartum providers who have trained in perinatal mental health disorders. Some midwives and OBGYNs will have training; some won't. It is worth your resources to find a provider that has been thoroughly trained.

Emily's Story

In our second session together, Emily sat on the couch in my office, her foot tapping against the carpet. Her baby was six weeks old, but she was alone today. I watched as she gripped the sleeve of her sweatshirt, pulling at a loose thread.

"I just . . . I don't know if I'm supposed to feel this way," she said quietly, staring at a spot on the rug that was beginning to fray.

I knew what was coming before she even said it. It was a line I'd heard so many times before—whispered in tearful confessions, blurted out in frustration, or barely audible beneath layers of shame.

"I love him, I really do . . . but I don't feel like myself. Shouldn't I be happy by now?"

Emily had given birth after a relatively smooth pregnancy. Her labor had been long but uncomplicated, and according to the photos she showed me, she and her baby were both healthy. On paper, everything was fine. And yet, here she was—expressing that she was unraveling, convinced that something inside her was broken because she wasn't radiating bliss.

"Everyone says it's the happiest time of your life," she continued. "But all I feel is . . . anxious. And numb. And sometimes I wish I could just disappear for a little while."

She immediately dropped her gaze, as if saying those words out loud made her unworthy of the title "mother."

I leaned forward slightly. "Emily, what if I told you that what you're feeling isn't a sign that something is wrong with you—but that you're adjusting to one of the biggest transformations a person can go through?"

Her eyes filled with tears. "But what if I never feel like myself again?"

It's a fear I've heard from so many women—this sense that the person they used to be is slipping away and they'll be left with someone lesser, someone permanently altered. What we don't talk about enough is that postpartum mental health is a spectrum—not a switch that flips the moment you meet your baby. It's entirely normal to feel grief alongside love, anxiety alongside joy, numbness alongside devotion.

"You're not supposed to feel like your old self," I told her gently. "Because you're becoming someone new. And that process takes time."

Over my years in private practice, I have always kept a list of psychiatrists that I work with. When a new client presents with the symptoms of a perinatal mental health disorder, I assure clients that I would never require medications, but I do encourage them to have an intake with a psychiatrist. Emily took the referral list and went ahead to schedule an intake with a wonderful psychiatrist. She had decided to explore medication management and had begun to take medications to help support her postpartum anxiety and depression.

Over the next few weeks, Emily continued to cry. She vented about the endless nights and the way the world seemed to expect her to bounce back when she could barely muster the energy to shower. We talked about intrusive thoughts—how common they are, even though no one warns you about them. We named things she hadn't dared to name yet—postpartum depression, identity loss, the loneliness of modern motherhood.

Slowly, her shoulders began to drop. She started texting her partner when she needed him to take over instead of powering through in silence. She asked her mom to come by in the afternoons so she could nap. She joined a new moms' group—even though she sat in the circle the first few times feeling like an outsider, waiting to feel something close to connection.

By the time her baby was four months old, she told me, "I'm still waiting to feel like myself again . . . but I think I'm starting to feel like *someone*."

That's what so many mothers are waiting to hear—that they're not broken, just becoming. That feeling like themselves might not be the goal at all, but instead, learning to meet the new version of themselves with curiosity instead of shame.

Perfect mental health doesn't exist—not in the postpartum period, not ever. But when we dismantle the myth that it should, we make space for something else: permission to struggle, to grieve, to feel joy in small, fleeting moments—and to trust that even in the mess, they are still becoming.

The History of Perinatal Mood Disorders

The earliest recorded case of postpartum mood disorders dates back to 700BCE, documented in the ancient Indian text "Charaka Samhita." This medical document describes a condition resembling postpartum depression, noting that some women, after childbirth, experience sadness, anxiety, and disinterest in daily activities. The text attributes these symptoms to imbalances in the body's vital energies and emphasizes the importance of family support and specific treatments to aid in recovery.

Similarly, ancient Greek physician Hippocrates, often referred to as the Father of Medicine, wrote about postpartum mood disturbances around 400 BCE. In his work Aphorisms, he mentions that "a woman is more liable to be seized with mania during puerperium," indicating an awareness of mood disorders following childbirth. Hippocrates believed these conditions were due to the retention of lochia (post-birth uterine discharge) and other bodily imbalances. His observations, though rooted in misconceptions of bodily fluids and humoral theory, highlight an enduring truth: the postpartum period has long been recognized as a vulnerable time for women's mental and physical health.

These early accounts demonstrate that postpartum mood disorders have been acknowledged and recognized across different cultures for a very long time, although interpretations and treatments have evolved over time. They also underscore the persistent challenge of distinguishing biological phenomena from societal expectations when studying women's reproductive health.

Have you ever heard of the theory of the wandering womb? If you were a woman in ancient Greece, it was believed that a woman's uterus wandered around her body to look for nourishment. Greek physicians used the idea of a wandering uterus to explain why women were so different from men. And for the Greeks, there was no ailment more dangerous for a woman than her womb wandering around her abdominal cavity.

To no surprise, the cure for a wandering womb was to keep women pregnant as often as possible to keep their womb occupied, and in its rightful place. Women were not only defined by their reproductive organs but also managed and controlled because of them. The idea of the wandering womb might sound absurd today, but the underlying narrative persists: the belief that a woman's primary purpose is reproduction and that any deviation from this norm is dangerous or defective.

Sound familiar? The woman is best kept at home, and the womb occupied so as to not start wandering.

Fast forward a few thousand years, and the myth of the wandering womb is gone—but its legacy remains. New moms are still up against the persistent myth that it's bad to have feelings outside of bliss and that the expression of sadness, anxiety, or anger makes us ungrateful or unfit. This societal pressure often leaves mothers feeling isolated and ashamed, particularly when they encounter postpartum mood disorders. The stigma is not only harmful but deeply entrenched, shaped by centuries of misunderstanding and judgment.

Today, we understand that postpartum mood disorders, including postpartum depression, anxiety and even psychosis stem from a complex interplay of hormonal changes, physical recovery and psychological adjustments. However, cultural narratives often oversimplify this experience, framing new motherhood as only a universally joyful time. This narrative leaves little room for the reality that most new moms face . . . an overwhelming fatigue, identity formation and the weight of a new responsibility.

Today, many mothers that are struggling with postpartum mood disorders avoid seeking support out of fear of being judged or misunderstood. Many worry that admitting to their struggles might lead to being labeled as unwell or bad, and accusation steeped in shame and surrounded with impossible to meet standards.

Women's bodies and mental health, particularly in the context of motherhood, have long been under-researched and misrepresented, or not represented at all in scientific literature, leading to gaps in knowledge that affect healthcare, policy and social perception. The lack of attachment has had profound implications for women, specifically with misdiagnosis and ineffective treatment options. Historical, social and structural factors have contributed to misinformation that influences how women's health, especially maternal mental health, is understood and treated.

For centuries, medical science treated male biology as the default, leaving women's health—and particularly maternal mental health—understudied and misunderstood. Until the 1990s, women were often excluded from clinical trials, and research on mental health relied on male-based diagnostic criteria, overlooking how pregnancy, childbirth, and hormonal changes shape women's experiences.

This neglect contributed to dismissive attitudes toward maternal mental health struggles, reducing conditions like postpartum depression to "baby blues" or personal weakness. The expectation that motherhood should feel intuitive and joyful only deepened the stigma, leaving many women isolated and without adequate care. While awareness has grown, research must continue to address not just biological factors but also the social and cultural pressures shaping maternal mental health.

What Can We Do?

In ancient texts, the recognition of postpartum struggles was paired with practical support—family involvement, prescribed rest, and treatments tailored to the individual. While these early interventions were rooted in the medical knowledge of their time, they reflected an important truth: moms thrive when they're supported (see chapter 7, wink wink). And so, what's the best way to move forward, armed with the tales of the past and medical knowledge of today?

First, we need to dismantle the myth of maternal bliss. It's essential to normalize the spectrum of emotions and experiences that accompany motherhood, from joy and love to fear and grief. Second, we advocate for systemic change that prioritizes maternal mental health. This includes improving access to postpartum care, providing paid family leave, and investing in community-based supports. These aren't luxuries; they're necessities that can significantly impact a mother's well-being and by extension, her family's health.

While it's important to honor the wisdom of the past while embracing the advances of the present, each can lend to each other to pave the way for supporting women during the postpartum period. Paving the way for a supportive period requires more than acknowledging what's broken—it calls for action. While systemic support may take time, there are immediate steps you can take to protect your well-being and build a more resilient foundation for your family. Enter the postpartum care plan: a practical tool designed to bring intention and support into the chaos of early parenthood. Let's explore how to create one that prioritizes your needs, fosters connection, and transforms the challenging first days into a more manageable and supported experience.

Signs to Watch for in Perinatal Mental Health

Perinatal mental health challenges—including depression, anxiety, and mood disorders—can begin during pregnancy or emerge after childbirth. While some emotional ups and downs are normal, certain signs indicate that a mother may need extra support. If you or someone you love is experiencing any of the following, it's important to seek help.

Emotional and Cognitive Signs can include:

- Persistent sadness, hopelessness, or feeling numb
- Intense guilt, shame, or feeling like a "bad mother"
- Racing thoughts, constant worry, or irrational fears
- Difficulty concentrating or making decisions
- Feeling disconnected from your baby or struggling with attachment

Physical and Behavioral Signs can include:

- Changes in sleep patterns (beyond typical newborn disruptions), such as insomnia or excessive sleeping
- Loss of appetite or overeating
- Fatigue that feels overwhelming, even when rested
- Frequent crying spells or feeling easily overwhelmed
- Withdrawal from loved ones or a lack of interest in activities once enjoyed

You might also experience:

- Thoughts of harming yourself or your baby. (You can visit earlier in this chapter where we chatted about intrusive thoughts, page 200.)
- Feeling like your baby or family would be better off without you
- Experiencing hallucinations, paranoia, or extreme confusion (which may indicate postpartum psychosis, a rare but serious condition requiring immediate medical attention)

If any of these symptoms persist for more than two weeks, intensify, or interfere with daily life, seeking professional support is crucial. Perinatal mental health struggles are common and treatable. You are not alone, and help is available.

Road Map to Change: Creating a Practical Guide to Support Your Perinatal Mental Health

Postpartum mood disorders are often misunderstood, minimized or ignored, leaving many moms to suffer in silence. But the truth is: maternal mental health is not a personal failing, but a collective responsibility. By shining a light on the complex realities of postpartum mood disorders, we can being to dismantle the stigma that keeps mothers isolated and unsupported.

Every mother deserves to feel seen, heard, and cared for—not just as a caretaker, but as an important, growing and whole person navigating one of life's most profound transformations. When we prioritize maternal mental health, we aren't just supporting mothers; we're creating healthier families, stronger communities, and a culture that values the well-being of all of its members.

The path through maternal mental health struggles aren't always easy, but healing is possible—with education, compassion and systems in place to support women in their transition into motherhood.

Small, intentional steps can make a significant difference. Here's a practical roadmap to support your well-being during this transition.

Roadmap to Change Exercises

A PRACTICAL GUIDE TO SUPPORTING PERINATAL MENTAL HEALTH

Perinatal mental health challenges can feel overwhelming, but small, intentional steps can help. Use this guide to care for yourself while adjusting to pregnancy and postpartum life. Each section includes reflection questions to help you check in with yourself along the way.

1. Build a Support System Before You Need It

- Identify a few trusted people (partner, family, friends) who can check in on you regularly.
- Join a local or online new parent support group.
- Set up practical support (meal trains, childcare help, housework assistance).

Reflection Questions

- Who in my life can I reach out to for emotional or practical support?
- Do I feel comfortable asking for help? If not, what's holding me back?
- What kind of support would make my daily life feel easier?

2. Prioritize Basic Needs

- Sleep: Take shifts with a partner or accept help for naps when possible.

- Nutrition: Keep easy-to-grab, nourishing snacks nearby. Eating regularly helps stabilize mood.
- Movement: Gentle movement (even a short walk outside) can improve mental health.

Reflection Questions

- Am I eating and drinking enough to sustain my energy?
- How can I improve my sleep, even in small ways?
- When was the last time I stepped outside or moved my body?

3. Set Realistic Expectations

- Lower the bar for housework and productivity—your well-being is the priority.
- Bonding takes time; don't pressure yourself to feel an instant connection.
- Remember that "good enough" parenting is what your baby needs—not perfection.

Reflection Questions

- What unrealistic expectations am I holding myself to?
- How would I treat a close friend in my situation?
- Can I give myself permission to let something go today?

4. Check In With Yourself Daily

Ask yourself:

- Am I feeling more down or anxious than usual?
- Am I able to enjoy moments with my baby, even briefly?
- Do I feel supported, or do I need to reach out for help?

Reflection Questions

- What emotions have been coming up most often for me?

- Have I been dismissing my feelings instead of addressing them?
- Is there someone I trust who I can share my thoughts with?

5. Communicate What You Need

- Be specific when asking for help ("Can you hold the baby while I nap?" instead of "I'm exhausted").
- Talk openly with your partner or a close friend about how you're feeling.
- Let visitors know what is (and isn't) helpful—sometimes just holding space is enough.

Reflection Questions

- Am I clearly communicating my needs, or am I assuming others will notice?
- What is one thing I wish people understood about what I'm experiencing?
- How can I practice being more direct about asking for help?

6. Seek Professional Help When Needed

- Know that postpartum depression and anxiety are common and treatable.
- Ask your ob-gyn or midwife about mental health screenings and referrals.
- Consider therapy, medication, or support groups—help comes in many forms.

Reflection Questions

- Have I been struggling with my mental health for more than two weeks?

- Do I feel like myself, or have I been feeling disconnected?
- What fears or hesitations do I have about seeking professional help?

7. Give Yourself Permission to Rest and Heal

- Motherhood is a major life shift—allow yourself time to adjust.
- Avoid comparing yourself to curated social media images of "perfect" motherhood.
- Remind yourself daily: You are not alone. You are doing enough. You deserve support.

Reflection Questions

- Am I judging myself harshly for struggling?
- What small act of self-compassion can I practice today?
- What would I say to a friend who was feeling the way I do?

You don't have to wait until things feel unbearable to ask for help. The earlier you acknowledge what you're experiencing, the sooner you can get the support you deserve.

Visit Appendix A: Postpartum Care Plan Worksheet (page 251) for an incredibly useful plan, with space to write, that will help you organize important dates, appointments, contact information. It will also help you plan ahead for what might happen during postpartum and will help you reflect on how you're feeling both physically and emotionally.

Three Important Things

1. If you experience a maternal mental health disorder, you are not broken; you are in need of very well deserved support.
2. It is okay to have conversations about your mental health with your provider at any time. It is their job to have supports in place for you.
3. Postpartum mood disorders are treatable, and there is no reason you have to suffer.

And what's next? Let's celebrate how amazing you are.

10

The Myth That Motherhood Isn't Ambitious

The myth that mothers can't be both ambitious and be great moms is not only outdated, but also harmful to all moms. It boxes women into a dichotomy where they are forced to choose between two core parts of their identity: the caregiver and the individual with goals and aspirations outside of motherhood. This binary denies the complexity of motherhood and the reality that ambition and parenting can, and often do, coexist beautifully.

When asked how I landed a literary agent, or a publishing deal, I usually say that I am motivated to create impact, that there is a huge need in the market for books that support postpartum moms, or that it's an extension of my clinical work but more accessible. Which are all true. I spent years telling myself, and others, that I had hustle, initiative, motivation and a knack for business. All those things are true, and all of those things are also another way of saying: I'm ambitious.

Yet, I've struggled to call myself ambitious, and I've never thought of myself as ambitious. I love my work, and I love being a mom. Job titles have never been important to me; instead, I'm motivated by supporting the well-being of those around me. My actions come from a genuine desire to help others—unsurprising, given that I'm a therapist. That said, if you looked at my career path on paper, you might describe me as an ambitious mom and woman.

Culturally, we become attached to the notion that if you want to be more than a mom, then you can't be a good mom. We've hammered into moms' brains that you have to pick one or the other: career success or parenting success. And the pressure to conform to this ideal is often intensified by society's narrow definition of ambition as being incompatible with good parenting.

Ambitious moms are often framed as selfish for prioritizing their own goals over their children. For women who have spent years perfecting their professional craft, working their way towards their work goals, it's unfair to assume they give it up when they become moms. Ambition, when applied to men and fathers, is praised as a sign of leadership, determination and strength. But when a mother is described as ambitious, the undertone is often negative, suggesting she's prioritizing her own success over their family's well-being.

This double standard is another one that reflects the cultural expectation that mothers must always put everyone else first, even at the expense of their own fulfillment. This narrative that glorifies mothers who give up everything—their careers, hobbies, and even personal time for the sake of everyone around them. While caregiving is undoubtedly a central part of parenthood, when we reduce a woman's identity only to caretaking, we miss so much of what a mom does and has to offer.

While caregiving is undoubtedly a central aspect of motherhood, this narrow definition overlooks the deeply ambitious nature of the role itself. Motherhood requires strategic thinking, long-term planning, adaptability, and the ability to foster growth and development in others. It is a profoundly ambitious undertaking, one that demands the same level of drive, vision, and leadership often celebrated in other areas of life. Mothers must continuously evaluate their children's needs, create opportunities for their development, and adapt to the ever-changing demands of each stage of life. They manage complex schedules, balance competing priorities, and make decisions with long-term implications. These are the hallmarks of ambition—setting a vision for the future and working diligently to bring it to life.

By redefining motherhood as an ambitious role, we can elevate its value and acknowledge the complexity and strength it requires.

Ambition and motherhood are not mutually exclusive. Pursuing personal goals can enrich a mother's life and, by extension, will benefit her children. A mother who is fulfilled, whether through her career, creative endeavors, motherhood itself or community involvement sets a powerful example for her kids. She shows them that it's possible to balance responsibilities and passions, to work hard for what you believe in, and to value your own growth alongside the care you give to others.

We must reframe ambition as something positive and deeply human, not as a trait that undermines motherhood. Ambition doesn't mean neglecting your family—it means honoring your whole self, including your personal and professional dreams. It means finding ways to integrate your own aspirations into the larger picture of your life, creating a family dynamic where everyone thrives.

Ambition is often viewed through a career-focused lens, associated with climbing corporate ladders, achieving professional milestones, or building businesses. Yet, ambition is much broader than these traditional markers. At its core, ambition is about striving for meaningful goals and embracing the challenge of growth. Motherhood embodies these principles in every sense. From the moment a woman becomes a mother, she embarks on a journey that requires her to set and pursue goals—for herself, her family and her life.

Ambition can take many forms, and it's not always tied to career milestones or climbing the corporate ladder. For some moms, ambition might look like turning a hobby into a business, going back to school, or. . . . writing a book. For others, it might mean cultivating a passion, volunteering in the community, or raising your voice on causes that you care deeply about. Whatever form it takes, ambition is not something that needs to be hidden or apologized for. It's something to embrace as part of a well-rounded and meaningful life.

The myth that you can't be ambitious and a good mom is rooted in fear—fear of breaking traditionally held molds, fear of judgment, and a fear of failure. But challenging this narrative and expanding our understanding of what motherhood can look like, we can empower moms to dream big, to take risks, and to pursue lives that reflect their whole selves. Because being a mom doesn't mean shrinking to fit someone else's expectations; it means growing into the fullest version of who you are.

Ambition isn't solely about external accomplishments; it's also about the internal work required to grow and evolve. Motherhood demands emotional ambition—the willingness to confront challenges, adapt to change, and nurture deep, meaningful connections.

Mothers often undergo a profound transformation as they navigate the complexities of parenthood. We have to learn to manage our own emotions while helping our children understand and process their own. We develop patience, resilience, and the ability to hold space for others to grow. These emotional skills are not innate; they are cultivated through hard work and determination, reflecting the nature of motherhood as ambitions.

Part of this reframing involves acknowledging the unique skills and strengths motherhood cultivates. Time management, conflict resolution, creative problem solving, and emotional intelligence. And those are only a few of the competence mothers develop. These skills are not only applicable to parenting but are also highly transferable in many other areas of our lives—community, career, relationships.

Instead of glorifying self-sacrifice as the ultimate marker of good mothering, we could honor the ambition it takes to raise children while striving for personal growth. This means celebrating the diverse ways mothers express their ambition, whether through career achievements, creative pursuits, community involvement or the deeply impactful work of parenting itself.

The implicit expectation that once a woman is a mother she should desire nothing outside of motherhood forces women to choose between their identity as mothers and their outside ambitions can make the pursuit of personal goals feel like an act of defiance.

Shortly after I became a licensed therapist, I started interviewing for new jobs. At the time, I was engaged and planning a wedding, but I didn't expect my personal life to become part of the interview process. During this interview with a male senior leader at a community mental health center, the conversation veered into uncomfortable territory. He began asking me questions about my wedding date and honeymoon plans. I remember feeling caught off guard and unsure of how to respond, especially since these questions seemed entirely unrelated to my qualifications for the role.

I was, at the very least, qualified for the position, meeting and exceeding both the educational and professional requirements listed. While being overqualified doesn't guarantee a job offer, it felt inappropriate for the interviewer to steer the discussion away from my skills and experience toward my personal life. Looking back, I'm pretty sure some of the questions he was asking me were illegal. Legally in the United States during an interview, you can't be asked if you're married, single, have children . . . any questions about your personal life that you aren't bringing up.

The experience left me feeling a little grossed out. Not just because of how inappropriate they were, but also about how women face such implicit biases through their careers. It seemed like a reminder of the subtle ways that gendered assumptions can influence professional opportunities.

Experiences like that interview revealed to me the unspoken barriers women face when navigating ambition alongside societal expectations of motherhood. There's an underlying assumption that a woman's personal life—her marriage, family plans, or status as a mom, undermines her professional abilities. And it shouldn't. What it really does is send the message that you can either excel in your career or embrace family life, but doing both makes you an exception, not the rule.

This myth—that being a good mom and pursuing personal or professional goals are mutually exclusive - has been repeatedly challenged by trailblazing moms throughout history.

A Timeline of Legal History of Women in The United States

When I take a step back and look at the bigger picture, I can see that for American women, ambition hasn't just been about rebellion. It's been about reclaiming power—the power to create the lives we want, rather than the ones we're told we should accept. Many women don't realize how recently these freedoms were won. It wasn't until the 1970s that women could even open their own credit cards, let alone allow themselves to dream of owning a business, leading a company or pursuing bold goals without permission.

And these victories didn't happen overnight. Generations of determined, ambitious women fought for every inch of progress that we have today. As you reach about these amazing women throughout this chapter, consider the legal milestone that made their achievements—and ours—possible.

- 1777: All states pass laws which take away women's right to vote.

- 1839: Mississippi becomes the first state to grant women the right to hold property in their own names without the permission of their husbands.
- 1866: The 14th Amendment is passed by Congress, with "citizens" and "voters" defined as male in the Constitution.
- 1873: The supreme court rules that a state has the right to exclude a married woman from practicing law.
- 1900: By this year, every state had passed legislation granting married women the right to keep their own wages and to own property in their own name.
- 1918: Two years after opening a birth control clinic in Brookly, Margaret Sanger's suit in New York allowed doctors to advise their married patients about birth control for health purposes. This clinic would become Planned Parenthood in 1942.
- 1920: The 19th Amendment is ratified, finally granting women the right to vote—but Jim Crow laws and other voter suppression tactics continue to disenfranchise Black women and other women of color.
- 1932: Hattie Wyatt Caraway, of Arkansas, becomes the first woman elected to the U.S. Senate.
- 1933: Frances Perkins becomes the first female cabinet member, appointed secretary of labor by President Franklin D, Roosevelt.
- 1963: The Equal Pay Act is passed by Congress, promising equitable wages for the same work, regardless of the race, color, religion, national origin or sex of the worker.
- 1965: The Supreme Court establishes the right of married couples to use contraception.

- 1973: Landmark Supreme Court ruling Roe v. Wade makes abortion legal.
- 1977: The Hyde Amendment is enacted, banning the use of federal funds for most abortion services, disproportionately impacting low-income women.
- 1978: The Pregnancy Discrimination Act bans employment discrimination against pregnant women.
- 1981: Sandra Day O'Connor becomes the first woman to serve on the Supreme Court.
- 1983: Dr. Sally K. Ride becomes the first American woman to be sent into space.
- 1992: Following the 1991 hearing in which lawyer Anita Hill accused Supreme Court nominee Clarence Thomas of sexual harassment, record numbers of women are elected to Congress, with four women winning Senate elections and two dozen women elected to first terms in the house.
- 1997: Madeleine Albright becomes the first female secretary of state.
- 2007: Nancy Pelosi becomes the first female speaker of the House.
- 2016: Hillary Rodham Clinton secures the Democratic presidential nomination, becoming the first U.S. woman to lead the ticked of a major party. She loses to Donald Trump.
- 2022: The Supreme Court overturns Roe v. Wade, the landmark case that established a right to an abortion nearly 50 years earlier.

These moments in history can serve to remind us that women's ambition has always been there, and has always served to challenge the status quo. Every achievement—whether it's working outside of the home, running for office, or balancing motherhood with career goals—builds on the progress of those who came before us. And every mom who dares to be ambitious today, even in the face of every hard moment, continues that legacy.

The Motherhood Tax

For many women, becoming a mother doesn't simply add a new layer to their identity; it subjects us to a unique set of societal and professional penalties, often referred to as the Motherhood Tax. The motherhood tax, also known as the motherhood penalty, is the economic and societal toll that women face after becoming mothers. Women with children earn less than women without children, even when they have similar education levels and occupations. On average, mothers make 63 cents for every dollar paid to fathers. Women with children may have fewer job opportunities and fewer chances for career advancement. And, mothers are viewed as less committed and less dependable employees, which could lead to hiring biases and lower job evaluation.

This often unspoken but tangible cost penalizes mothers in most areas of life outside of parenthood, creating significant barriers in our careers, finances and overall wellness. To navigate this, many mothers feel an immense pressure to overcompensate—to work hard, prove their worth and justify their successes in spaces where the dual roles of mother and employee are scrutinized.

And, the Motherhood Tax isn't just theoretical; it's backed by research and in the stories of many moms who had the lived experiences. Everything from wage gaps to slower career progression and fewer opportunities for leadership roles after having children. A landmark study by sociologists Shelley Correll, Stephen Benard and In Paik found that mothers were viewed as less competent and committed than their child-free peers. In hiring scenarios, mothers have been offered lower starting salaries, fewer promotions and harsher evaluations despite identical qualifications.

Though more women than ever are entering and excelling in the workforce, society hasn't fully adjusted its expectations. The "ideal worker" archetype remains deeply masculine—a person who is available 24/7, unencumbered by caregiving duties. When mothers enter professional spaces, their dual role conflicts with this archetype. Their need for flexibility or accommodation is viewed not as a necessity but as evidence of a lack of commitment. The message is clear: pick one—career or motherhood.

In response to the Motherhood Tax, many women internalize the need to overcompensate. They overperform at work, striving to prove that they can "do it all" without missing a beat. They stay late, overcommit to projects, and answer emails at all hours to make up for the stigma of going on leave to have a baby. Many working mothers describe this overcompensation as an exhausting but necessary survival tactic—a way to secure their place in a system that sees their dual role as a liability.

For example, a mother who returns to work after parental leave often feels the need to jump right back in—return to work like she never had a baby and return home like it's her fulltime job. She worries that any sign of struggle—whether it's fatigue, adjusting to a new routine, or asking for accommodations—would confirm negative stereotypes. To counter this, she may push herself harder, take on more tasks, or work with poor boundaries even if it compromises her well-being. This relentless effort is less about ambition and more about survival—a way to prove she's not slacking at work or distracted by her role as mom.

And this same pressure may also extend beyond the workplace. Socially, mothers face an impossible standard: they must be fully present at work while simultaneously being the perfect mom at home. A working mom who takes pride in her career may still feel the pressure to compensate for her time away by overperforming as a mother—planning elaborate birthday parties, volunteering at school, preparing homemade meals, and being constantly available to her family. It's a performance of perfection, rooted in the fear of being judged.

The emotional toll of the motherhood tax and overcompensation is profound. Mothers experience burnout, anxiety, self-consciousness, feelings of failure, internalized pressure and the fear of falling short in all areas of their lives.

Neutralizing the stigma around ambition requires a cultural shift in how we define and talk about it. Ambition does not have to be synonymous with greed, cutthroat behavior, or neglecting family values. Instead, it can be reframed as a positive quality—one rooted in personal fulfillment, growth, and the desire to contribute meaningfully to society. Ambition can reflect a mom's passion for her work, her dreams of creating financial security for her family, or her hope to leave the world better for her children. When we celebrate ambition as an expression of purpose and joy rather than a rejection of traditional maternal ideals, we allow space for moms to embrace their full identities without guilt or shame.

Ambitious Moms I Love

Representation and storytelling matter. By highlighting the stories of ambitious moms—those who have pursued careers, built businesses, or made significant contributions to their communities while loving their children fiercely—we begin to challenge the narrative. Women like Ruth Bader Ginsburg, Michelle Obama, and Elizabeth Warren demonstrate that ambition and motherhood are not mutually exclusive but can fuel one another. Their successes provide a new framework for mothers to see ambition as something worth striving for, not something to apologize for. Ambition doesn't diminish a mother's love or commitment to her children; rather, it models resilience, passion, and the courage to dream big.

After becoming a mom to Malia and Sasha, **Michelle Obama** masterfully balanced motherhood with impactful achievements - hi, she was a lawyer and then built the most gorgeous garden at the White House. As First Lady, she prioritized her daughters' stability amidst the demands of public life, maintaining family routines and creating a grounded environment. Obama launched the Let's Move campaign to combat childhood obesity, Joining Forces to support military families, and Reach Higher to inspire youth to pursue higher education. In 2018, Obama published her memoir, *Becoming*, which became a global bestseller. Post-White House, she continued her advocacy through the Obama Foundation, focusing on leadership development and empowerment.

After becoming a mom to her two children, **Ruth Bader Ginsburg** achieved groundbreaking accomplishments that transformed the legal landscape for gender equality. Balancing motherhood with her ambitions, she often credited her family responsibilities with teaching her time management and focus, skills that fueled her success. As a young mother, Ginsberg attended Harvard law School, where she excelled despite being one of the only few women in the class. She went on to found the Women's Rights Project at the ACLU in 1970. In 1993 she became the second woman appointed to the U.S. supreme court, where she championed equality, civil rights and justice for nearly three decades.

Judith Love Cohen was an American aerospace engineer. She was an electrical engineer on the Minuteman missile, the science ground station for the Hubble Space Telescope, the Track and Data Relay Satellite and the Apollo Space Program. She is credited with helping save Apollo 13 with her work on the Abort-Guidance System. On the day that she went into labor with her fourth child, Judith was troubleshooting problems with schematics. The baby that was born while she problem solved saving Apollo 13 was who we know as the actor and musician Jack Black.

Maya Angelou became a mother to her son, Guy, at the age of 17. Angelou achieved extraordinary accomplishments that cemented her as a literary icon and cultural leader. Despite the challenges of single motherhood, she pursued a wide-ranging career with determination, always crediting her role as a mother as the central source of her strength and inspiration. Her 1969 memoir, *I Know Why the Caged Bird Sings*, became a groundbreaking work, shedding light on issues of race, identity and resilience. Later in her life, she became a celebrated teacher, speaker, writer and the ultimate storyteller.

After becoming a mother, **Dolores Huerta** achieved groundbreaking success as a labor leader and civil rights activist. She was the co-founder of the United Farm Workers alongside Cesar Chavez and she played a pivotal role in advocating for the rights of farmworkers, often bringing her children to organizing. Her leadership was instrumental in securing better wages and working conditions for ag laborers. Beyond her work with the UFW, Huerta spent decades advocating for women's rights, immigrant rights, and education reform. Even as a mother, she worked tirelessly to mentor young activists.

Each of these women, at some point, had the choice to decide between ambition and family, and they all chose both. Stories like theirs are exactly what modern moms need to hear to start neutralizing the stigma around the word ambition, and what it means to be an ambitious mom.

Your Personal Definition of Ambition

Not every woman will—or should—pursue traditional career ambition, and that's equally valid. The goal is to create a culture where women feel free to define their aspirations on their own terms without judgment. Whether a mom stays home, starts a business, or works a demanding job, her choices should be respected and valued. By reclaiming ambition as a term of empowerment rather than critique, we can begin to dismantle the barriers that keep mothers from owning their desires and showing up fully—both for their families and themselves.

Celebrating individual choices means recognizing that no single path to fulfillment fits everyone and that each mother's journey is deeply personal. It's about valuing that every woman has the agency to decide what feels right for her life, whether that involves pursuing a high-powered career, staying home to raise her children, or carving out a unique balance between the two. When we focus on personal agency over rigid identities, we allow women the freedom to define success on their own terms without fear of judgment.

This shift not only validates diverse experiences of motherhood but also acknowledges that ambition can look different for everyone. For some, it might be chasing professional dreams; for others, it could mean mastering the art of caregiving or championing a cause close to their heart. By honoring these choices as equally worthy, we create a culture where women feel empowered to embrace their whole selves—mothers, dreamers, creators, and everything in between.

For generations, women have faced immense societal pressure to see motherhood as the pinnacle of their aspirations - career or otherwise, often at the expense of their other dreams, talents, and ambitions. The truth, however, is that motherhood can be a part of your ambition—a big, beautiful part—or it can be the centerpiece of your life. Either way, there is no wrong choice. The important thing is that the decision reflects your personal values and desires, not the expectations of others.

For some women, the role of "mom" is central to how they see themselves. They find great fulfillment in devoting their time, energy, and talents to raising children, nurturing their families, and building a home. Choosing to make motherhood their primary focus is not a sign of limitation or a lack of ambition—motherhood in itself is the most ambitious act steeped in love and dedication. This decision is often accompanied by societal criticism, where women are sometimes undervalued or dismissed as "just a mom," as though raising the next generation is anything less than monumental. It's crucial to honor and celebrate those who find joy and purpose in making motherhood the cornerstone of their identity.

On the other hand, for many women, motherhood is just one facet of who they are. They may feel equally drawn to their careers, creative pursuits, hobbies, or causes they're passionate about. They might find purpose and fulfillment in contributing to their communities, innovating in their fields, or expressing themselves outside the realm of parenting. These mothers are often scrutinized under the lens of societal judgment that questions their commitment to their children simply because their identity extends beyond the home. But being a mother doesn't mean you stop being a person with your own dreams, goals, and aspirations. In fact, showing children that moms are complex, multidimensional people can be a powerful lesson.

The notion that a woman must choose between being a good mother and ditching any hobbies, interests or careers outside of family creates a false binary. Women who prioritize motherhood aren't necessarily surrendering their individuality, just as women who pursue personal ambitions aren't neglecting their role as mothers. It's not about having it all or choosing one path over the other—it's about having the freedom to decide what balance works best for you in different seasons of life. For some, motherhood may become more central during certain life phases, while other parts of their identity take precedence at other times.

What matters most is giving women the space to define their own paths. We must challenge the idea that there's a "right way" to mother or a single standard of what a fulfilling life looks like. Some women thrive when motherhood is their primary focus, while others feel alive when balancing parenting with their passions and pursuits outside the home. Both approaches are valid, and both deserve respect.

Ultimately, the conversation isn't about choosing motherhood over personal identity or vice versa. It's about recognizing that every woman has the agency to decide how she wants motherhood to shape her life. Whether a woman sees motherhood as her ultimate calling, part of a rich tapestry of roles, or anything in between, the choice is hers to make. Let's celebrate that individuality and honor the diversity of ways women define themselves.

Road Map to Change: Your Ambition Audit

Whether your dreams include professional success, creative expression, community involvement, or simply being fully present with your children, there is no "right" way to balance it all. The key is crafting a life that feels authentic to you, honoring both your role as a mom and your personal ambitions in a way that aligns with your unique values.

It's also important to embrace the fluidity of identity. What feels right for you today might evolve as your children grow, as your career shifts, or as your interests deepen. Give yourself the grace to explore these changes without guilt or judgment.

Whether motherhood becomes your main passion, a facet of your identity, or something in between, it is your choice—and that choice is inherently valid. By accepting this truth, you can release the pressure to fit a predefined mold and instead focus on creating a fulfilling, balanced, and joyful life on your own terms.

Roadmap to Change Exercises

It's easy to feel torn between the nurturing role of raising children and the ambitions that fuel your personal and professional growth. This exercise is designed to help you explore the intersection of these two identities by clarifying your values, defining your goals, and visualizing how motherhood and ambition can coexist in harmony. Through reflection and intention, this worksheet empowers you to embrace your multifaceted identity and create a life that honors both your family and you.

Take time to reflect on each section below. Answer as honestly as possible, knowing that this is a judgment-free space for self-discovery.

UNDERSTANDING YOUR CORE VALUES

Your values shape your decisions and help build meaning. Reflect on the principles that guide you.

1. What values matter most to you? (examples: compassion, growth, independence, creativity, family)
2. How do you see these values reflected in your role as a mom?
3. How do these values influence your ambitions outside of motherhood?

EXPLORING YOUR GOALS

Goals provide direction and motivation. This section will help you clarify what you want to achieve in both motherhood and your personal pursuits.

1. Write down three personal or professional goals you are working towards.
2. Write down three hopes or intentions you have for your experience in motherhood.
3. How can these goals and intentions support each other rather than compete?

EXAMINING THE INTERSECTION OF MOTHERHOOD AND AMBITION

Finding harmony between parenting and personal ambition involves identifying overlaps and reducing friction.

1. What unique strengths has motherhood brought to your personal and professional life?
2. What challenges do you face in balancing your ambitions with Motherhood?
3. Name one area where motherhood and your ambition complement each other.

Visualizing Your Ideal Identity

This section invites you to imagine the future version of yourself that integrates your values, goals and roles seamlessly.

1. Describe the mom you want to be (your parenting identity).
2. Describe the professional or personal individual you want to be (your ambition identity).
3. What does an ideal day look like where these two identities can exist in balance with each other?

Action Plan: Bridging the Gap

Turn your reflections into concrete steps to align your motherhood and your ambition.

1. List one small habit or routine you can create to support your parenting values.
2. List one small habit or routine you can create to support your personal or professional goals.
3. Identify a support system or resource that can help you manage these roles.

YOUR GUIDING MANTRA

Combine your reflections into a guiding mantra—a phrase or sentence that inspires you to embrace your happiest balance.

Example: "I am a nurturing mom and a driven woman; my values guide me to create a life of meaning and purpose.

Write your mantra here:

____

Take a moment to review your answers. What insights has this exercise helped you clarify?

Three Important Things:

1. Motherhood is an ambitious act.
2. Your version of motherhood doesn't have to look like anyone else's; you get to make it what you want.
3. You are allowed to have an identity that is multifaceted, complex, dynamic and authentic to you.

What's coming next? I leave you with this question: where do we go from here?

You're Already Changing the World, Promise

Hopefully, by the time you've reached this moment, you have had a lot of "oh hell yes!" or *very loud therapeutic exhale* moments, you are feeling clearer in your path and feeling a lot more ok with being anything less than perfect.

Before I get too sappy, I would love to say from the deepest parts of my heart, I am so honored to be mothering alongside you. You and I are raising our future leaders, the next generation of caregivers—our futures are forever enmeshed, and I am grateful for that. When you choose to share your gifts with the world, you are helping to make a better future for all of us. I'm lucky to have you, your baby is lucky to have you, and in the long history of mothers—this time in history is lucky to have you and every gift you bring to it.

Throughout this book, we've explored the myths that have shaped our understanding of early motherhood, and how, for generations, women have been burdened by unrealistic expectations and societal pressures. We've delved into the ways these myths—about instant attachment, the "right" way to feed a baby, or the ideal mother—have misled us, making us feel isolated, inadequate, or as if we're failing. Yet, at the heart of every myth is a fundamental truth: there is no singular way to be a mother, and every mother's journey is valid.

The freedom to define what motherhood means for you is one of the most empowering choices you can make. This book is not just about debunking myths, but about reclaiming the space to make motherhood your own. There is no right or wrong way to mother—whether motherhood becomes your ultimate calling, a vibrant part of your life alongside other passions, or something you balance with career and personal pursuits, the decision is yours to make.

I'm often asked what my favorite tips and tricks are for conquering postpartum with confidence and ease. And the answer is two-fold:

1. There is no trick for conquering postpartum - it's a stage with a deep learning curve that all new moms must go through. It will be easier for some than for others, but please remember that we will all have parts we are challenged by. There is no such thing as postpartum and perfection.
2. Postpartum isn't a problem that needs to be solved. And if that's how you are experiencing it, I encourage you to scratch the surface of that belief and explore which part of you is wanting solutions - I'd guess it's the perfectionism part of you.

In the midst of COVID in 2020, I was experiencing postpartum for a second time, and a short time later I launched 4th Trimester Wellness on Instagram. Moms were lonely. Moms were isolated. And I wanted to offer even the smallest bit of validation and support. And then, a 4th Trimester Wellness Survival Guide that I had created, but was too hesitant to do anything with made it to an editor at Hallmark, who put me in touch with a consultant who had worked as an acquisitions editor. She read over my work and said, "You can self-publish this, or you can traditionally publish this, I think either way it's a really important resource." This was the beginning of 2022.

It took me an entire year, from the end of 2022 to the end of 2023, to work through my "I'm not a writer, I'm just a mom and a therapist" self-doubt. And at the end of it, I had read every book about writing books, had made a list of my top five literary agents, had completed my proposal and query letter and told my husband, "I'm going to send this to five agents. If I get an agent, great. If not, I learned a lot and I'll move on." I sent out 5 queries in December 2023, and had signed with my agent in January of 2024. From June 2024 to December 2024, I wrote this book. While working, and parenting, and maintaining my marriage, starting a podcast, moving to a new city.

New moms, stay at home moms, career pausing moms, single moms, adoptive moms and every variation in between, please don't discount your "cute little idea" as unattainable. Please don't let your imposter syndrome keep you from dreaming. Please don't let little hiccups in your mental health or hard feelings be the reason you stop trying. Please don't let your fear of being imperfect steal a life's worth of beautiful moments. Beyond the desire for perfection exists a place where you allow yourself to reach the goals that you have for yourself, your kids, your family.

I was recently sitting with my daughter as she was playing with her dolls. One doll was telling her another doll, "I'm writing a book just like my mommy." Our kids are so smart, they see everything. When we are able to be our most authentic and true selves, we are teaching our kids to do the same.

The first time I ever said out loud, "I want to write a book for new moms, everyone talks about the baby, why aren't we talking about being a mom?" my daughter was still in the NICU. Discovering and understanding the stories we've been told, the stories we've absorbed, our own stories and myths around perfection and the idea of postpartum being easy has changed the course of parenting for me, and hopefully it has for you as well.

If you take only one thing from this book, let it be this: you already have everything you need to be the mom you are meant to be. I promise.

Postpartum isn't meant to be perfect, but we're also not here to be perfect; that isn't our purpose. If we hold on tightly to the reigns of perfection, we stop growing in any meaningful way. And becoming a mom isn't the end of one thing, but the beginning of a whole new stage. Honor it. Reflect on it. Celebrate it. Imperfections and all.

In the end, the myth of a perfect postpartum experience only serves to add pressure to an already challenging time. The truth is that motherhood—especially in the postpartum period—is inherently imperfect, and that imperfection is where the beauty lies. By embracing the messiness, the unpredictability, and the bumps along the way, you create space for real moments of joy and connection with yourself, your baby, and your family.

Rather than striving for an unattainable ideal, focus on what feels right for you. Let go of the comparison, the shame, and the guilt that come with trying to measure up to an unrealistic standard. Instead, build a new reality—one that's rooted in authenticity, acceptance, and compassion for yourself. The joy of the postpartum period isn't found in perfection, but in the small, everyday moments that remind you of your strength, resilience, and capacity to love.

So, let's redefine what postpartum joy looks like—not as a flawless picture, but as an imperfect journey that's uniquely yours. Embrace it with open arms, and know that every step, no matter how messy, is part of your beautiful, unfolding story.

As you close this book, I want to tell you that I'm really proud of you. You've challenged the myths, unpacked the pressures, and embraced the reality that there's no one-sized-fits-all version of motherhood. You've learned to trust yourself, honor your needs, and redefine what it means to be a mother on your own terms. Now, take what your mama gave you and go gift it to yourself, your kids and the world. We need your sparkle. There is no perfect version of motherhood—there is only your version. And that's exactly what the world needs.

APPENDIX A

Postpartum Care Plan Worksheet

The purpose of a postpartum care plan is to proactively organize and address the needs of a new parent during the earliest days of parenthood. By mapping out resources, supports, and strategies in advance, this plan ensures that new parents are not left to navigate postpartum alone.

This care plan is a living document—update it as your needs and circumstances change. Remember: asking for help is an act of strength, not weakness. You deserve care and support during this transformative time.

Feel free to write your answers directly in the book or copy this plan to your journal. Note that at the end, I provide questions meant for you to answer weekly. Feel free to answer those in a journal.

1. Immediate Postpartum Recovery

A. Physical Recovery

- **Rest and Sleep Preferences:**
  - o How will you prioritize sleep?

    ____

    ____

- Who can help with nighttime care?

  ____

- **Nutrition Plan:**
  - What types of meals/snacks will you have ready?

    ____

    ____

    ____

    ____

    ____

  - Who can assist?

    ____

    ____

- **Hydration Strategy:** How will you ensure access to water throughout the day?

  ____

  ____

- **Postpartum Check-ups:** When are your scheduled appointments?

  ____

  ____

  ____

  ____

  ____

- **Healing Supplies:** List any items you plan to use (e.g., perineal spray, belly band):

  ____

  ____

  ____

  ____

  ____

  ____

  ____

___

___

___

B. Emotional Recovery

- **Daily Emotional Check-Ins:** How will you track your mood?

___

___

- **Mental Health Resources:** List contacts for therapists, crisis hotlines, or support groups

___

___

___

___

___

2. Parental Leave and Visitors

- **Parental Leave Schedule:** Write down start and end dates for each parent.

___

___

- **Visitor Preferences:** Who will visit, and when? Are there any boundaries you'd like to set?

___

___

___

- **Visitor Support Plan:** How can visitors contribute (e.g., bring meals, help with household tasks)?

___

___

___

3. Infant Care Support

A. Feeding Plan

- **Preferred Feeding Method(s):** (Breastfeeding, formula feeding, or combination):

  ____

- **Lactation Consultant Contact (if applicable):**

  ____

- **Formula Supplies Needed (if applicable):**

  ____

  ____

B. Sleep Support

- **Safe Sleep Setup:** (e.g., crib, bassinet location):

  ____

- **Nighttime Routine Ideas:**

  ____

  ____

  ____

4. Household Management

A. Delegating Responsibilities

- **Partner Role:** What tasks will your partner take on?

  ____

  ____

  ____

  ____

  ____

- **Family/Friend Support:** Who can help with specific tasks (e.g., meals, errands)?

  ____

  ____

  ____

- **Professional Help:** Will you hire cleaning services, meal delivery, or childcare? If so, which ones?

____

____

B. Organized Supplies

- Where will you keep essential items (e.g., diapers, feeding supplies)?

____

____

5. Social and Emotional Connection

A. Support Network

- **List of Supportive People (Friends, Family, Groups):**

____

____

____

____

____

____

____

____

____

____

- **Parenting Groups:** Online or in-person groups to join:

____

____

____

____

____

- **Workplace Support Contact (if applicable):**

____

B. Self-Care

- **Activities That Recharge You:** (e.g., a walk, reading, mindfulness exercises):

- **Personal Care Rituals:** How will you make time for daily care?

6. A Sleep and Rest Plan

- **Daily Rest Goals:** How will you fit rest into your day?

- **Nighttime Assistance Plan:** Who will handle night-time feedings or diaper changes?

- **Nap Strategies:** When and where can you nap during the day?

7. Sibling and Pet Support

A. Older Sibling Care

- **Daily Routine:** What activities will help older siblings adjust?

- **Support Network:** Who can assist with sibling care (e.g., grandparents, friends)?

____

____

- **Special Time:** How will you ensure one-on-one time with older siblings?

____

____

B. Pet Care

- **Feeding and Walk Schedule:** Who will take care of your pet's needs?

____

- **Vet Contact:** List your veterinarian's contact info:

____

____

- **Emergency Plan:** Who can take care of your pet if needed?

____

____

8. Community Support

- **Local Resources:** What community groups or services are available to you?

____

____

- **Postpartum Doula Contact (if applicable):**

____

____

- **Faith-Based or Cultural Organizations:**

____

____

____

9. **Mental Health Support**
    - **Therapist or Counselor Contact:**

      ____

      ____

    - **Signs to Watch For:** What symptoms might indicate you need additional support?

      ____

      ____

      ____

      ____

      ____

    - **Crisis Plan:** Who will you call if you need immediate help?

      ____

      ____

10. **Return to Work and Partner Return to Work**
    - **Parent's Return-to-Work Plan:** Timeline and adjustments needed:

      ____

      ____

    - **Partner's Return-to-Work Plan:** How will their return impact household tasks?

      ____

      ____

    - **Childcare Arrangements:** What plans are in place for childcare?

      ____

      ____

    - **Workplace Communication:** What flexibility or support can you request?

      ____

      ____

11. Long-Term Postpartum Health

A. Postpartum Check-Ins

- **Physical Healing Progress:** Notes/concerns:

  ____
  ____
  ____
  ____
  ____

- **Emotional Well-Being:** How are you feeling day-to-day?

  ____
  ____
  ____
  ____
  ____

- **Feeding Goals:** Progress and any changes:

  ____
  ____
  ____
  ____
  ____

B. Returning to Exercise

- **Preferred Activities:** (e.g., walking, yoga):

  ____
  ____
  ____
  ____
  ____

Clearance from Healthcare Provider: Date:

____

C. Sexual Health

- **Discussion with Provider:** Notes/concerns:

12. Customizing Your Plan

A. Cultural or Religious Practices

- List any rituals or traditions you'd like to incorporate:

B. Personal Preferences

- What specific needs do you have for your postpartum period?

Weekly Check-In Questions

1. How am I feeling physically?

2. How am I feeling emotionally?

3. What support do I need from others this week?

4. Are there any appointments or follow-ups I need to schedule?

5. Am I making time for self-care, even in small ways?

APPENDIX B

Additional Resources for Your Postpartum Journey

We know that motherhood is a profound transition—one that is as complex as it is deeply personal. While this book has explored many of the myths and challenges that shape early motherhood, the conversation doesn't end here. Whether you're looking for more in-depth reading, expert guidance, or supportive communities, this appendix offers a curated list of books and organizations that provide valuable insights and resources for new mothers.

From evidence-based postpartum care to personal stories of navigating the fourth trimester, these recommendations are here to remind you that you're not alone. No matter where you are in your journey—whether you're struggling with intrusive thoughts, adjusting to your new identity, or simply looking for reassurance—there are resources to support you. Take what resonates, leave what doesn't, and know that your experience of motherhood is uniquely yours to shape.

Motherhood, Postpartum Health and Mental Health

- *Matrescence: On the Metamorphosis of Pregnancy, Childbirth, and Motherhood*—Lucy Jones
- *And Now We Have Everything: On Motherhood Before I Was Ready*—Meaghan O'Connell

- *What No One Tells You: A Guide to Your Emotions from Pregnancy to Motherhood*—Alexandra Sacks & Catherine Birndorf
- *Good Moms Have Scary Thoughts*—Karen Kleiman
- *Dropping the Baby and Other Scary Thoughts*—Karen Kleiman & Amy Wenzel
- *It's Not Hysteria: Everything You Need to Know About Your Reproductive Health (but Were Never Told)*—Dr. Karen Tang

Relationship Support & Parenting After Baby

- *How to Not Hate Your Husband After Kids*—Jancee Dunn
- *Fight Right: How Successful Couples Turn Conflict Into Connection*—Julie Schwartz Gottman PhD and John Gottman PhD
- *Where Should We Begin: The Arc of Love* - Esther Perel
- *Parenting from the Inside Out: How a Deeper Self-Understanding Can Help You Raise Children Who Thrive*—Daniel J. Siegel & Mary Hartzell
- *Raising Securely Attached Kids: Using Connection-Focused Parenting to Create Confidence, Empathy, and Resilience (Attachment Nerd)*—Eli Harwood
- *The Whole-Brain Child: 12 Revolutionary Strategies to Nurture Your Child's Developing Mind*—Daniel J. Siegel & Tina Payne Bryson

Healing from Trauma & Personal Growth

- *The Body Keeps the Score*—Bessel van der Kolk
- *Adult Children of Emotionally Immature Parents: How to Heal from Distant, Rejecting, or Self-Involved Parents*—Lindsay Gibson
- *It Didn't Start with You: How Inherited Family Trauma Shapes Who We Are and How to End the Cycle* by Mark Wolynn

- *No Bad Parts: Healing Trauma and Restoring Wholeness with the Internal Family Systems Model* by Richard Schwartz
- *The Deepest Well: Healing the Long-Term Effects of Childhood Trauma and Adversity* by Nadine Burke Harris

Postpartum Nutrition & Hormonal Health

- *The First Forty Days*—Heng Ou

Organizations & Resources for Moms
Maternal Mental Health & Postpartum Support

- Postpartum Support International (PSI)—www.postpartum.net
- The Motherhood Center—www.themotherhoodcenter.com
- National Maternal Mental Health Hotline—1-833-9-HELP4MOMS
- March of Dimes (Postpartum Recovery & Health)—www.marchofdimes.org

Feeding Support

- La Leche League International—www.llli.org
- The Infant Risk Center (Medications & Breastfeeding Safety)—www.infantrisk.com

Parenting & Relationship Resources

- Gottman Institute (Marriage & Parenting Research)—www.gottman.com
- Attachment Parenting International—www.attachmentparenting.org
- Zero to Three (Early Child Development)—www.zerotothree.org

ACKNOWLEDGMENTS

Being a therapist can, at times, be a very solitary profession. So much of the work I've done as a therapist has existed in a terrarium. It's sealed and vibrant and maintained. Therapists set up safe and secure environments where everything that steps in can grow. And growth isn't just for the clients; there is growth in this space for the therapist as well. So first and foremost, I owe my thanks to everyone along the way that has helped sustain my growth both personally and professionally. Mentors, teachers, clients, group members, peers, physicians and other therapists.

At the heart of my growth—and growing right alongside me—is my husband, Richie. When I first toyed with the idea of writing a book for new moms, our kids were just 2 and 4. Richie has moved mountains to make this possible, and there aren't enough ways to thank him. Without him, this book wouldn't exist. And, of course, without him, there wouldn't be a Jack and Ruby.

I had no way of knowing that becoming a mom would completely change the trajectory of my life. There's the parenting itself, but also the unexpected way motherhood has become a gateway to doing the work I love—something I never could have predicted.

First, there is no way I would be able to have done this without my kids, Jack and Ruby. Without them, there would be no mom/Erin/author combination. Jack, you are earnest, you cry from happiness, you are beautiful, inclusive, kind, funny, loving and your curiosity will change the world. Ruby, you are hilarious, determined, you love to celebrate life, you are tiny and fierce, loving, smart, beautiful and wise. Your spirit will change the world.

You are my favorite little people, even though I haven't slept in 8 years. Thank you Richie, Jack and Ruby for being encouraging, non-judgmental, creating space and giving me grace, encouraging me, loving me and being honest with me when it's time to take a break.

I can't imagine my life without the three of you, truly. Life is endlessly more meaningful because each of you are in it. I love you Richie, I love you Jack and I love you Ruby. I love doing life with you.

To my literary agent Amanda Bernardi, you took a chance on me, and I am so grateful that you did. One of the first times Amanda and I met, she was in a coffee shop with sick kids and I was home with sick kids. It was a match made in parenting heaven. She showed up, I showed up, and I knew working with her could make magic. I also knew that this was the singular person who would understand and work to amplify my voice and all postpartum moms access to support. Amanda was told that postpartum moms don't read, and she charged ahead with this project knowing that this book would be exactly what many new moms need. Also to note, postpartum moms read. You advocated for me, supported me as a first time author AND always seem to remain calm and collected. A true queen.

To my Editor Laura Apperson, you also took a chance on me, and again, I am so incredibly grateful. Right after meeting for the first time I told my husband "I adore the editor I met with today, she was wearing overalls her husband bought her and I have a feeling that she's going to be a mom before this book comes out." And, as I'm writing this, Laura is in the final stages of pregnancy before welcoming her first baby. I feel so honored that our lives collided at this exact time, while we are both preparing to embark on new and unknown paths. Also, to any aspiring writers, GET LAURA ON YOUR TEAM. She's an incredible editor, and she also plays flute—like could she be any cooler?

And a special thanks to my mom, my dad and my in-laws, this work surely would have been left incomplete if it wasn't for your support. Both in supporting and encouraging me, and helping with Jack and Ruby for the sake of book writing. I feel really really lucky to be surrounded by such loving support and I am forever grateful that we all live within three minutes of each other. And to my sister, Sarah, who is my best friend. There is nobody else I would want to talk to 400 times a week through the ups and downs of life and love and motherhood.

BIBLIOGRAPHY

Abramowitz, Jonathan S., Sarah A. Schwartz, Katherine M. Moore, and Kelly R. Luenzmann. "Obsessive-Compulsive Symptoms in Pregnancy and the Puerperium: A Review of the Literature." *Journal of Anxiety Disorders* 17, no. 4 (2003): 461–78.

American College of Obstetricians and Gynecologists. "Committee Opinion No. 757: Screening for Perinatal Depression." *Obstetrics and Gynecology* 130, no. 5 (2017): e208–e212.

American Medical Association. "How the Use of BMI Fetishizes White Embodiment and Racializes Fat Phobia." *Journal of Ethics*, July 2023. https://journalofethics.ama-assn.org/article/how-use-bmi-fetishizes-white-embodiment-and-racializes-fat-phobia/2023-07.

Aristotle. *Politics*. Translated by C. D. C. Reeve. Indianapolis: Hackett, 1998.

Arms, Suzanne. *Immaculate Deception: A New Look at Women and Childbirth in America*. Houghton Mifflin, 1975.

Aquinas, Thomas. *Summa Theologica*. Translated by Fathers of the English Dominican Province. Benziger Bros., 1911.

Bailey, Zinzi D., Nancy Krieger, Madina Agénor, et al. "Structural Racism and Health Inequities in the USA: Evidence and Interventions." *The Lancet* 389, no. 10077 (2017): 1453–63. https://doi.org/10.1016/S0140-6736(17)30569-X.

Ban Zhao. "Lessons for Women (Nüjie)." Translated by Patricia Ebrey. In *Sources of Chinese Tradition*, Vol. 1, edited by Wm. Theodore de Bary and Irene Bloom, 826–31. Columbia University Press, 1999.

Bipolar Village (website). http://www.bipolarvillage.com/2015/05/.

Blum, Linda M. *At the Breast: Ideologies of Breastfeeding and Motherhood in the Contemporary United States*. Beacon Press, 1999.

Brockington, Ian. *Motherhood and Mental Health*. Oxford University Press, 1996.

Brown, Brené. *The Gifts of Imperfection: Let Go of Who You Think You're Supposed to Be and Embrace Who You Are*. Hazelden, 2010.

Buckley, Sarah J. *Hormonal Physiology of Childbearing: Evidence and Implications for Women, Babies, and Maternity Care*. Childbirth Connection Programs, National Partnership for Women and Families, 2015. https://pubmed.ncbi.nlm.nih.gov/26834435/.

Budig, Michelle J., and Paula England. "The Wage Penalty for Motherhood." *American Sociological Review* 66, no. 2 (2001): 204–25.

Bureau of Labor Statistics. "Employment Characteristics of Families—2023." April 2024. https://www.bls.gov/news.release/pdf/famee.pdf.

Cahill, Heather A. "Male Appropriation and Medicalization of Childbirth: The Contribution of the Male Gynaecologist in the Nineteenth Century." *Journal of Advanced Nursing* 33, no. 3 (2001): 334–42.

Caraka, Avinash Chandra. *Charaka-Samhita*. Translated into English. Calcutta: Caraka, 1890–1914.

Carter, Pam. *Feminism, Breasts and Breast-Feeding*. Macmillan, 1995.

Cleveland Clinic. "Body Changes During Pregnancy." Last reviewed May 2022. https://my.clevelandclinic.org/health/articles/9682-body-changes-during-pregnancy.

Cleveland Clinic. "Postpartum Recovery: What to Expect." https://health.clevelandclinic.org/postpartum-recovery.

Confucius. *The Analects*. Translated by Arthur Waley. Macmillan, 1938.

Connor, Thomas G., Thomas G O'Connor, Catherine Monk, and Elizabeth Fitelson. "Practitioner Review: Maternal Mood in Pregnancy and Child Development—Implications for Child Psychology and Psychiatry." *Journal of Child Psychology and Psychiatry and Allied Disciplines* 55, no. 2 (2014).

Cook, A., M. Blaustein, J. Spinazzola, and B. van der Kolk, eds. *Complex Trauma in Children and Adolescents*. Guilford Press, 2003.

Correll, Shelley J., Stephen Benard, and In Paik. "Getting a Job: Is There a Motherhood Penalty?" *American Journal of Sociology* 112, no. 5 (2007): 1297–339. https://doi.org/10.1086/511799.

Deci, Edward L., and Richard M. Ryan. "The 'What' and 'Why' of Goal Pursuits: Human Needs and the Self-Determination of Behavior." *Psychological Inquiry* 11, no. 4 (2000): 227–68.

Dennis, Cindy-Lee, and Lori Ross. "Women's Perceptions of Partner Support and Conflict in the Development of Postpartum Depressive Symptoms." *Journal of Advanced Nursing* 56, no. 6 (2006): 588–99.

Dick-Read, Grantly. *Childbirth Without Fear: The Principles and Practice of Natural Childbirth.* Harper & Brothers, 1944.

Drife, J. "The Start of Life: A History of Obstetrics." *Postgraduate Medical Journal* 78, no. 919 (May 2002): 311–5. doi: 10.1136/pmj.78.919.311.

Dunne, J., K. Rebay-Salisbury, R. B. Salisbury, A. Frisch, C. Walton-Doyle, and R. P. Evershed. "Milk of Ruminants in Ceramic Baby Bottles From Prehistoric Child Graves." *Nature* 574, no. 7777 (2019): 246–48.

Ebers Papyrus. *The Ebers Papyrus: A New English Translation, Commentaries and Glossaries.* Translated by Paul Ghalioungui. Cairo: Academy of Scientific Research and Technology, 1987. https://meretsegerbooks.cld.bz/ghalioungiebers.

Eleftheriou, Georgios, Georgios Eleftheriou, Raffaella Butera, et al. "Consensus Panel Recommendations for the Pharmacological Management of Breastfeeding Women With Postpartum Depression." *International Journal of Environmental Research and Public Health* 21, no. 5 (2024): 551.

Farrow, Michelle. *Embracing Radical Acceptance and Letting Go of Control.* Mind Shift Therapy & Neurofeedback. July 30, 2024. https://www.mindshifttherapy.ca/post/embracing-radical-acceptance-and-letting-go-of-control.

Erikson, Erik H. *Identity and the Life Cycle.* W. W. Norton, 1959.

Fairbrother, Nichole, and Sheila R Woody. "New Mothers' Thoughts of Harm Related to the Newborn." *Archives of Women's Mental Health* 11, no. 3 (2008): 221–9.

Federal Reserve Board. *Report on the Economic Well-Being of U.S. Households in 2023.* May 2024. https://www.federalreserve.gov/publications/2024-economic-well-being-of-us-households-in-2023-executive-summary.htm.

Feldman, Ruth, Ilanit Gordon, and Orna Zagoory-Sharon. "Maternal and Paternal Plasma, Salivary, and Infant Oxytocin and Parent-Infant Synchrony: Considering Stress and Affiliation Components of Human Bonding." *Developmental Science* 14, no. 4 (July 2011), 752–61. doi: 10.1111/j.1467-7687.2010.01021.x.

Fernandez, Jennifer, and Rose Hoban. "Lawmakers Look to Address Maternal Mortality Gaps." *The Charlotte Post* 49, no. 34 (2023): 1B.

Field, Tiffany. "Postpartum Depression Effects on Early Interactions, Parenting, and Safety Practices: A Review." *Infant Behavior and Development* 33, no. 1 (2010): 1–6. https://doi.org/10.1016/j.infbeh.2009.10.005.

Fildes, Valerie A. *Wet Nursing: A History From Antiquity to the Present.* Basil Blackwell, 1988.

Fox-Genovese, Elizabeth. *Within the Plantation Household: Black and White Women of the Old South.* University of North Carolina Press, 1988.

Gavin, Nancy I., Bernard Z. Gaynes, Karen N. Lohr, et al. "Perinatal Depression: A Systematic Review of Prevalence and Incidence." *Obstetrics and Gynecology* 106, no. 5 (2005): 1071–1083. https://doi.org/10.1097/01.AOG.0000183597.31630.db.

Glynn, Laura M, Elysia Poggi Davis, Curt A Sandman, and Wendy A Goldberg. "Gestational Hormone Profiles Predict Human Maternal Behavior at 1-Year Postpartum." *Hormones and Behavior* 85 (2016): 19–25.

Gordon, Ilanit, Orna Zagoory-Sharon, James F. Leckman, and Ruth Feldman. "Oxytocin and the Development of Parenting in Humans." *Biological Psychiatry* 68, no. 4 (2010): 377–82.

Harlow, Harry. "Total Social Isolation in Monkeys." *Proceedings of the National Academy of Sciences of the United States of America (1965).* Accessed August 5, 2024. https://www.ncbi.nlm.nih.gov/pmc/articles/PMC285801/pdf/pnas00159-0105.pdf.

Harvard Health Publishing. "Body Image and Mental Health." Harvard Medical School. Accessed December 10, 2024. https://www.health.harvard.edu.

Hewlett, Sylvia Ann. *Off-Ramps and On-Ramps: Keeping Talented Women on the Road to Success.* Harvard Business Review Press, 2007.

Hochschild, Arlie Russell. *The Second Shift: Working Families and the Revolution at Home.* Penguin Books, 2012.

Hollingworth, Leta S. "Social Devices for Impelling Women to Bear and Rear Children." *American Journal of Sociology* 22, no. 1 (1916): 19–29. http://www.jstor.org/stable/2763926.

Karp, Harvey. *The Happiest Baby on the Block: The New Way to Calm Crying and Help Your Newborn Baby Sleep Longer.* Bantam Books, 2003.

Kessel, David. "The Birth of Anesthesia: Queen Victoria's Role in the Acceptance of Chloroform." *British Medical Journal* 330, no. 7488 (2005): 730–731.

Kim, Sohye, and Lane Strathearn. "Oxytocin and Maternal Brain Plasticity: Implications for Postpartum Depression and Bonding." *New Directions for Child and Adolescent Development*, no. 153 (September 2, 2016): 59–72. doi: 10.1002/cad.20170.

Leavitt, Judith Walzer. *Brought to Bed: Childbearing in America, 1750–1950*. Oxford University Press, 1986.

Levine, Peter A., and Maggie Kline. *Trauma Through a Child's Eyes: Awakening the Ordinary Miracle of Healing*. North Atlantic Books, 2007.

Levy, Terry M., and Michael Orlans. *Attachment, Trauma, and Healing: Understanding and Treating Attachment Disorder in Children and Families*. Jessica Kingsley, 1998.

Loudon, Irvine. *Death in Childbirth: An International Study of Maternal Care and Maternal Mortality, 1800–1950*. Clarendon Press, 1992.

Marcia, James E. "Development and Validation of Ego Identity Status." *Journal of Personality and Social Psychology* 3, no. 5 (1966): 551–58.

Mayo Clinic. "Postpartum Depression." Last modified June 2021. https://www.mayoclinic.org/diseases-conditions/postpartum-depression/symptoms-causes/syc-20350927.

Mayo Clinic. "Pregnancy Week by Week." Accessed November 2024. https://www.mayoclinic.org/healthy-lifestyle/pregnancy-week-by-week/expert-answers/pregnancy-body-changes/faq-20058072.

Mayo Clinic Staff. "Self-Esteem Check: Too Low or Just Right?" Mayo Clinic. Last modified May 12, 2022. https://www.mayoclinic.org.

McAdams, Dan P. 1996. "Personality, Modernity, and the Storied Self: A Contemporary Framework for Studying Persons." *Psychological Inquiry* 7 (4): 295–321. doi: 10.1207/s15327965pli0704_1.

Mercer, Jean. *Understanding Attachment: Parenting, Child Care, and Emotional Development*. Praeger, 2006.

Meeussen, Loes, and Colette Van Laar. "Feeling Pressure to Be a Perfect Mother Relates to Parental Burnout and Career Ambitions." *Frontiers in Psychology* 9 (November 4, 2018). https://www.frontiersin.org/journals/psychology/articles/10.3389/fpsyg.2018.02113/full.

Morgan, Jennifer L. *Laboring Women: Reproduction and Gender in New World Slavery*. University of Pennsylvania Press, 2004.

Murthy, Vivek H. *Parents Under Pressure: The U.S. Surgeon General's Advisory on the Mental Health and Well-Being of Parents*. Washington,

DC: U.S. Department of Health and Human Services, August 2024. Accessed May 23, 2025. https://www.hhs.gov/surgeongeneral/reports-and-publications/parents/index.html.

National Institute of Mental Health. "Perinatal Depression." https://www.nimh.nih.gov/health/publications/perinatal-depression.

Neff, Kristin D. *Self-Compassion: The Proven Power of Being Kind to Yourself.* HarperCollins, 2011.

Neumark-Sztainer, Dianne. *I'm, Like, SO Fat! Helping Your Teen Make Healthy Choices About Eating and Exercise in a Weight-Obsessed World.* Guilford Press, 2005.

Numan, Michael and Thomas Insel. *The Neurobiology of Parental Behavior.* Springer Science & Business Media, 2003.

O'Hara, Michael W., and Annette M. Wisner. "Perinatal Mental Illness: Definition, Description, and Aetiology." *Best Practice and Research Clinical Obstetrics and Gynaecology* 28, no. 1 (2014): 3–12. https://doi.org/10.1016/j.bpobgyn.2013.09.002.

Osterman, Michelle J. K., and Joyce A. Martin. "Trends in Low-Risk Cesarean Delivery in the United States, 1990–2013." *National Vital Statistics Reports* 63, no. 6 (November 5, 2014). https://www.cdc.gov/nchs/data/nvsr/nvsr63/nvsr63_06.pdf#:~:text=The%20overall%20cesarean%20delivery%20rate%20in%20the,be%20delivered%20by%20cesarean%20every%20year%20(2).

Raphael, Dana. *The Tender Gift: Breastfeeding.* Schocken Books, 1973.

Rousseau, Jean-Jacques. *Émile, or On Education.* Translated by Allan Bloom. Basic Books, 1979. Originally published 1762.

Sacks, Alexandra. *What No One Tells You: A Guide to Your Emotions From Pregnancy to Motherhood.* Simon & Schuster, 2019.

Sacks, Alexandra. "The Birth of a Mother." *The New York Times*, May 8, 2017. https://www.nytimes.com/2017/05/08/well/family/the-birth-of-a-mother.html.

Schroeder, Fred E. H. "The Secret History of Menstruation." *JSTOR Daily*, February 20, 2023. Accessed October 23, 2024. https://daily.jstor.org/the-secret-history-of-menstruation/.

Schwartz, Marie Jenkins. *Birthing a Slave: Motherhood and Medicine in the Antebellum South.* Harvard University Press, 2006.

Simon, Matt. "Fantastically Wrong: The Theory of the Wandering Wombs That Drove Women to Madness." *Wired*, May 7, 2014. https://www.wired.com/2014/05/fantastically-wrong-wandering-womb/.

Simpson, James Young. *The History of Chloroform and Other Anesthetics*. Adam and Charles Black, 1858.

Stevens, Emily E., Tonse N. K. Raju, and Kiran P. Southall. "History of Wet Nursing: A Journey From Ancient to Modern Times." *Journal of Perinatology* 28, no. 4 (2008): 334–39.

Stevenson, Brenda E. *Life in Black and White: Family and Community in the Slave South*. Oxford University Press, 1996.

Substance Abuse and Mental Health Services Administration. Table 3.13, "DSM-IV to DSM-5 Obsessive-Compulsive Disorder Comparison." In *Impact of the DSM-IV to DSM-5 Changes on the National Survey on Drug Use and Health*. Available from https://www.ncbi.nlm.nih.gov/books/NBK519704/table/ch3.t13/.

Tajfel, Henry, and John C. Turner. "An Integrative Theory of Intergroup Conflict." In *The Social Psychology of Intergroup Relations*, 33–47. Brooks/Cole, 1979.

U.S. Department of Health and Human Services. "Surgeon General's Advisory: The Mental Health Crisis Among Parents." August 2024. Accessed March 23, 2025. https://www.hhs.gov/surgeongeneral/reports-and-publications/parents/index.html.

Vicedo, Marga. "The Social Nature of the Mother's Tie to Her Child: John Bowlby's Theory of Attachment in Post-War America." *British Journal for the History of Science* 44, no. 3 (2011): 401–26. http://www.jstor.org/stable/41241684.

Warner, Judith. "The Myth of the Perfect Mother." *Newsweek*, February 21, 2005.

Welter, Barbara. "The Cult of True Womanhood: 1820–1860." *American Quarterly* 18, no. 2, part 1 (Summer 1966): 151–74.

Wertz, Richard W., and Dorothy C. Wertz. *Lying-In: A History of Childbirth in America*. Yale University Press, 1989.

West, Emily, and R. J. Knight. "Mothers' Milk: Slavery, Wet-Nursing, and Black and White Women in the Antebellum South." *Journal of Southern History* 83, no. 1 (2017): 37–68. https://dx.doi.org/10.1353/soh.2017.0001.

Wickes, Igor Grant. "A History of Infant Feeding: Part II. Seventeenth and Eighteenth Centuries." *Archives of Disease in Childhood* 28 (1953): 232–40. doi: 10.1136/adc.28.139.232.

Wolf, Jacqueline H. *Deliver Me From Pain: Anesthesia and Birth in America*. Johns Hopkins University Press, 2009.

INDEX